AIDS: Social Representations, Social Practices

AIDS: Social Representations, Social Practices

Edited by

Peter Aggleton, Graham Hart and Peter Davies

Routledge
Taylor & Francis Group
LONDON AND NEW YORK

First published 1989 by Routledge Falmer

Published 2016 by Routledge
2 Park Square, Milton Park, Abingdon, Oxfordshire OX14 4RN
711 Third Avenue, New York, NY 10017

First issued in paperback 2016

Routledge is an imprint of the Taylor and Francis Group, an informa business

Library of Congress Cataloging-in-Publication Data

available on request

British Library Cataloguing in Publication Data

AIDS: social representations, social practices.
1. AIDS. Social aspects.
I. Aggleton, Peter, 1952– II. Hart, Graham.
III. Davies, Peter.
362.1′042.

ISBN 1-85000-430-7
ISBN 1-85000-431-5 (pbk.)

Typeset in 11/13pt Bembo by
Photo·graphics, Honiton, Devon

Jacket design by Caroline Archer

ISBN 13: 978-1-138-96641-3 (pbk)
ISBN 13: 978-1-85000-430-1 (hbk)

CONTENTS

Preface vii
Acknowledgements viii
Chapter 1 AIDS: The Intellectual Agenda
Jeffery Weeks 1
Chapter 2 One Epidemic or Three? Cultural, Social and Historical Aspects of the AIDS Pandemic
Ronald Frankenberg 21
Chapter 3 Undergraduates' Beliefs and Attitudes About AIDS
Stephen Clift and David Stears 39
Chapter 4 The Subject of AIDS
Simon Watney 64
Chapter 5 Perverts, Inverts and Experts: The Cultural Production of an AIDS Research Paradigm
Meyrick Horton with Peter Aggleton 74
Chapter 6 Making Sense of a Precipice: Constituting Identity in an HIV Clinic
David Silverman 101
Chapter 7 Gay Men's Sexual Behaviour in Response to AIDS – Insights and Problems
Ray Fitzpatrick, Mary Boulton and Graham Hart 127
Chapter 8 Some Notes on the Structure of Homosexual Acts
Peter Davies 147
Chapter 9 HIV and the Injecting Drug User
Graham Hart 160

Chapter 10	Methods of Drug Use: Injecting and Sharing *Robert Power*	173
Chapter 11	Syringe-Exchange Schemes in England and Scotland: Evaluating a New Service for Drug Users *Gerry V. Stimson, Lindsey Alldritt, Kate Dolan and Martin Donoghoe*	186
Chapter 12	Injecting Drug Use and HIV Infection – Intervention Strategies for Harm Minimization *Geraldine Mulleady, Graham Hart and Peter Aggleton*	199
Chapter 13	Marginalized Groups and Health Education About HIV Infection and AIDS *Tina Wiseman*	211
Chapter 14	Evaluating Health Education About AIDS *Peter Aggleton*	220
Chapter 15	Resistance and the Erotic *Cindy Patton*	237
Chapter 16	Reading AIDS *Jan Zita Grover*	252
Notes on Contributors		264
Index		267

Preface

In November 1987, the second UK Conference on Social Aspects of AIDS took place at the Polytechnic of the South Bank in London. This brought together a wide range of researchers with an interest in examining the social dimensions of HIV infection and AIDS. Amongst those present were educationalists, psychologists, sociologists and anthropologists, as well as representatives from statutory and voluntary sector organizations providing services for those affected by AIDS.

This book contains many of the papers given at the conference as well as a number of additional contributions. In editing it, we have been conscious of the need to document the kind of research that is currently taking place as well as opportunities for future enquiry. We would like to thank all those who attended the conference for their courage and commitment in these difficult times. In particular, we must express our gratitude to Paul Broderick, Adrian Coyle, Miriam David, Hilary Homans, Andrew Hunt, Debbie Lowry, Paul Simpson and Kaye Wellings who played a key role in planning and organizing the conference. We also owe a special debt to AVERT (AIDS Education and Research Trust) for their financial support. Finally, we must thank Helen Thomas who prepared the manuscript for publication.

Peter Aggleton, Graham Hart and Peter Davies
June 1988

Acknowledgements

The chapter 'Resistance and the Erotic' by Cindy Patton was originally published in *Radical America*, 20, 6, pp. 68–74. The chapter 'The Subject of AIDS' by Simon Watney was originally published in *Copyright*, 1. Both of these chapters are reproduced with permission.

1
AIDS: The Intellectual Agenda

Jeffrey Weeks

All diseases have social, ethical and political dimensions. Diseases affect individuals, not abstract entities or collectivities, and affects them in variable ways, according to their general social condition and bodily health. What makes disease culturally and historically important, however, is the way in which meanings are attached to illness and death, meanings and interpretations which are refracted through a host of differing, and often conflicting and contradictory social possibilities. These shape the ways we interpret illness, and therefore organize the ways in which we respond.

There is a long tradition of connecting disease with moral issues: 'sickness' and 'sin' are terms which have long been linked, and often interchangeably, especially in periods of heightened social anxiety. So there is nothing intrinsically new in the ways in which AIDS has been culturally interpreted, signified and given strong moral meaning. Some time ago, Susan Sontag famously deplored the tendency for illness to become a metaphor — a process whereby the specifics of individual suffering are lost in a welter of social fantasy (Sontag, 1983; Alcorn, 1988). More recent historical studies have shown that sex-related diseases have gained a particularly powerful grip on the social imagination: in nineteenth-century England, for example, syphilis became known as the 'social disease', while its supposed source of infection, prostitution, was known as the 'social evil' (Weeks, 1988a).

At the same time, other diseases became the bearers of sexual meanings. Frank Mort's recent book *Dangerous Sexualities* (Mort, 1987) has demonstrated very clearly that at least from the early nineteenth century responses to epidemics of various types have been shaped by a host of moral assumptions about the sexual behaviour of those they affected. These assumptions insensibly infiltrate medical theories and responses, and in turn shape and reshape popular attitudes. Illnesses such as cholera and typhoid, TB and cancer, have all carried a heavy burden of moral anxiety, and have attained a massive symbolic significance, because attempts have been consistently made to link individual failings (especially with regard to sex), social marginality, and moral inadequacy with a tendency to acquire one or other of them.

In one sense then the social response to AIDS has been governed by the same tendency to moral inflation that has characterized a number of other life-threatening diseases in the past. But there are also important differences, differences which reveal much about the times we are living in. In the first place we are living through *this* disease, and the ways in which it is affecting us, and people we know and love, and the communities we inhabit. Second, we are living in a culture which at one time seemed to promise the triumph of technology over the uncontrollable whims of nature, and yet here is a new virus that has apparently confounded science. As Neil Small put it, 'The impact of AIDS is essentially linked with modernity — its virulence and relative untreatability lead us to question a cornerstone of faith in science, experts and progress' (Small, 1988).

Third, and perhaps most important, AIDS has become the symbolic bearer of a host of meanings about our contemporary culture: about its social composition, its racial boundaries, its attitudes to social marginality; and above all, its moral configurations and its sexual mores. A number of different histories intersect in and are condensed by AIDS discourse. What gives AIDS a particular power is its ability to represent a host of fears, anxieties and problems in our current, post-permissive society.

My aim in this chapter is not so much to provide an exhaustive explanation of why this is the case as to offer an intellectual framework within which we can identify the main forces at work. I shall begin by identifying the main phases of the social reaction to AIDS this far in its history. Through this it will be possible to characterize the present. Put briefly, my argument will be that AIDS already has a complex history which irrevocably shadows the way we think and the way we act. I will then discuss some of the key issues that need to be addressed in responding to the AIDS crisis. These provide the outlines of an agenda for historical and social science research, and for the political and social approaches needed to live with AIDS.

Responses to AIDS

Looking back over the years since 1981, when AIDS first emerged as a new and devastating illness, there is a potential danger that we will see the period as a monolithic whole, characterized by a deepening crisis and geometric spread of the disease. Emotionally, certainly, it sometimes feels like that, and in a sense recent political responses are based on the premise that only a deepening crisis could justify the actions that governments are now beginning to take. But it is not ultimately useful to try to understand the history of AIDS in these terms. There have, in fact, been at least three distinct phases in the social responses to AIDS so far. The boundaries between these are neither clear cut, nor absolute. Many features recur throughout, though with different weightings and emphases. Nevertheless, each period has its own distinct characteristics. Each needs looking at in turn.

The Dawning Crisis (1981–82)

There is of course a pre-history to AIDS stretching back to the mid-1970s, and by 1980 the dimensions of the potential crisis were already beginning to appear in statistics recording health problems amongst gay men (Shilts, 1988). It was not until the summer of 1981, however, that these developments became an embryonic public issue. It was then that the first stories began to appear in medical journals and in the gay press reporting the emergence of mysterious new illnesses among gay men in the USA. There were three major features of this first phase.

First, there was an awakening sense of anxiety amongst those most immediately affected, mainly gay men in the American cities with large gay populations (New York, San Francisco and Los Angeles), but also members of the Haitian community in America, and haemophiliacs. At the same time, this was accompanied by a certain moral and sexual complacency which suggested that this new illness was either a scare story or a minority problem. This was the period when gay men began debating whether they needed to change their sexual habits, when fears began to emerge about the possible effects of AIDS on the achievements of gay liberation, and when those who advocated sexual abstinence or safer sex (for example, Berkowitz and Callen, 1983) were denounced for delivering the lesbian and gay community back into the embrace of the medical discourse from which it had all too recently escaped (Weeks, 1985). Because the cause, or causes, of the syndrome of illnesses were unknown, so the responses were contested and confused.

Second, there were exploratory medical and scientific attempts to define the nature, epidemiology and significance of this new phenomenon. These can be traced in the evolution of the terminology used to describe the syndrome – from 'the gay cancer' to GRID (Gay-Related Immune Deficiency), to the eventual acceptance in 1982 of the acronym AIDS – a shift, at least in the scientific world, from the initial identification of the disease with the community that first experienced it to a recognition of a more general danger. The four Hs were rapidly identified as 'risk categories': homosexuals, heroin users, haemophiliacs and, most controversially of all, Haitians. Allied to this shift were certain problems. Too narrow a definition of AIDS, relating it only to its terminal stages, threatened to encourage the view that the illness was invariably fatal, and resistance to it hopeless. But too broad a definition, to cover all of what became known as AIDS related conditions and the presence of sero-positivity, threatened equally to obscure important distinctions. Alongside these debates, feeding them and confusing them, was the beginnings of a highly competitive and personally poisonous race to identify the cause of AIDS, and find a cure — a race tainted by the lure of Nobel laureates, high prestige and profits (McKie, 1986; Shilts, 1988).

Third, this period saw the development of the characteristic style of governmental response that was to dominate the next phase: widespread indifference. There were many factors influencing this, including the coincidence that in the USA, and to a lesser extent elsewhere, the onset of AIDS occurred at the very moment that the Federal Administration was intent on cutting public expenditure. But over and above this, there was the overwhelming fact that AIDS was a disease that seemed to be confined to marginal, and (with the possible exceptions of haemophiliacs) politically and morally embarrassing, communities. More particularly, it was seen as a gay disease at a time when the view was being sedulously cultivated that the gay revolution had already gone too far (Weeks, 1986 and 1989).

Moral Panic (1982–1985)

The marginality of people with AIDS, and its identification as a 'gay plague', were central to the second phase which occurred between

1982–85, that of moral panic. Moral panics occur in complex societies when deep rooted and difficult to resolve social anxieties become focused on symbolic agents which can be easily targetted. Over the past century sexuality has been a potent focus of such moral panics — prostitutes have been blamed for syphilis, homosexuals for the cold war and pornography for child abuse and violence. Whilst the concept of a moral panic does not explain why transfers of anxiety like these occur — this has to be a matter for a historical analysis — it nevertheless offers a valuable framework for describing the course of events (Weeks, 1985; and for a critique of moral panic theory see Watney, 1987 and 1988).

From about 1982, AIDS (now identified as a distinctive set of diseases with definable, if as yet not precisely known, causative factors), became the bearer of a number of political, social and moral anxieties, whose origins lay elsewhere, but which were condensed into a crisis over AIDS. These included issues such as 'promiscuity', permissive lifestyles and drug taking. In this particular context, Paula Treichler has made the point that whilst safer sex might protect us from the virus, it can not protect us from this expanded meaning of 'AIDS', which now becomes a potent symbolic agent in its own right (Treichler, 1987).

This period of moral panic was characterized by a number of features. First, it saw the rapid escalation of media and popular hysteria. This was the golden period of the New Right and Moral Majority onslaught in the USA, with leading lights claiming to see in AIDS God's or nature's judgment on moral decay. This was the period also when the term 'gay plague' became the favourite term of tabloid headline-writers (Wellings, 1988). This was the time when people with the disease were blamed for it. These were the years which witnessed the widespread appearance of 'rituals of decontamination': lesbians and gay men were refused service in restaurants, theatre personnel refused to work with gay actors, the trash cans of people suspected of having AIDS were not emptied, children with the virus were banned from schools, and the dead were left unburied. 'AIDS' as a symbolic phenomenon thereby grew out of, and fed into, potent streams of homophobia and racism.

Second, during 1983 and 1984, despite rather than because of the frantic international rivalry, the Human Immunodeficiency Virus (HIV) was at last identified and given its agreed name. This opened new opportunities for responding to the disease; but it also, inevitably, signalled the formidable difficulties in producing a vaccine against it, or a cure for it.

Third, this period saw the emergence of a massive self-help response from the communities most affected, and particularly from the lesbian and gay community. Organizations such as Gay Men's Health Crisis in New York or the Terrence Higgins Trust in London emerged as much more than special interest pressure groups. They became, in the absence of a coherent national strategy, the main vehicles of health education and social support. As Robert Padgug (1986) has suggested, one of the most striking features of AIDS has been the unusual, perhaps unique degree to which the group that was most affected by it took part in all aspects of its management. This included the provision of social aid and health care to people with AIDS, whether gay or not, the conduct of research, lobbying for funds and other government intervention, the creation of educational programmes, and negotiation with legislators and health insurers.

While governments throughout the West remained largely silent, these self-help groupings achieved remarkable results in safer-sex education. The identification of the virus, and its likely modes of transmission, made it clear that it was wrong to talk of risk categories; there were instead *risk activities*. And risk itself could be reduced by relatively simple measures — by using condoms, by cutting out certain unprotected sexual activities, and by not sharing needles if you were an injecting drug user. What was needed above all was education on prevention. Whilst national governments were as yet reluctant to undertake this, others by necessity picked up the candle, and with notable success too. By 1984, to take one example, 95 per cent of gay men in San Francisco knew how AIDS was transmitted and knew the risk guidelines. To take another, sexually transmitted disease rates amongst gay men began to drop significantly as safer sex guidelines were codified and made readily available (Small, 1988). This was almost entirely due to work within the lesbian and gay community itself.

Crisis Management (1985 to the present)

1985 was the turning point. Partly this was a result of chance factors, the most important of which was the well publicized illness and death of Rock Hudson which dramatized the impact of the disease, and the inadequacy of American facilities: Hudson went to Paris, where in fact the virus had first been isolated, for treatment. The major reason, however, was the increasing evidence that AIDS was not just a disease of execrated minorities but a health threat on a global scale, and one which in world terms, largely affected heterosexuals. This initiated the period in which we now live, one in which the dominant response has been crisis management.

There are a number of key characteristics of this period. First, governments began to respond on a scale that approximated a little more to the magnitude of the crisis. As Randy Shilts has reminded us, by the time President Reagan had delivered his first speech on AIDS, six years into the crisis, over 36,000 Americans had been diagnosed with the syndrome, and some 20,000 had died (Shilts, 1988). From 1985, however, we can trace a new urgency in governmental response. In Britain there had been virtually no government response until 1984. Only then was there intervention to prevent the further contamination of the blood supply (and by implication, prevent the spread of AIDS to 'the innocent'). In 1985, the government took powers compulsorily to detain in hospital people who were perceived as likely to ignore medical advice and were at risk of spreading the disease. Both these measures were dictated by a fear that AIDS might infiltrate the so-called general population. But in 1985 only £135,000 was set aside by the government for education and prevention. By the end of 1986, with the dramatic adoption of a new policy in November of that year, this had leapt a hundredfold (Weeks, 1986b).

This change of heart was not the result of a sudden excess of altruism. The key factor was the generalization of risk, and the key precipitating event came with the publication of the US Surgeon-General's report on AIDS in October 1986. This allowed AIDS to achieve the 'critical mass' to become a major issue on the official social agenda (Shilts, 1988).

The new policy was organized around a sustained public campaign aimed at preventing the spread of the virus — this is the second major characteristic of the period. There was a certain historical irony therefore in the fact that the shift in policy was inspired by an arch-conservative Reaganite appointee in the USA (the Surgeon-General, Dr. C.E. Koop), and led by the Thatcher government in Britain at a time when its moral agenda reasserting traditional family values, rolling back the tide of 'permissiveness', and sharply defining the limits of sex education in schools, was unfolding. For a policy of prevention aimed not only to warn the general population about the risks, but to work with, and to take advantage of experience generated within the very lesbian and gay community it elsewhere sought to challenge (Weeks, 1988).

A third characteristic flowed from this shift in policy, accentuating trends already in existence: the period witnessed a significant 'professionalization' of organized responses to AIDS. In part, this involved a professionalization of the self-help groupings themselves, as public funds flowed into them, and demands upon their services increased. A new alliance, not without its problems, between the medical profession and the communities at risk began to be forged. At the same time, a different sort of professionalism began to emerge which actively distanced itself from the lesbian and gay community as AIDS became seen as a universal problem. Moreover, as Silverman points out elsewhere in this book, as a consequence of HIV, genito-urinary medicine and allied medical practice moved from being cinderella specialisms to well-funded, high status work.

As if by a necessary reflex, this period also saw the rapid growth of alternative health care and therapies, as people with AIDS and HIV infection have sought to retain responsibility for the condition of their own bodies (Spence, 1986; Tatchell, 1986).

Finally, the period has seen a deepening of the health crisis itself, as the dimensions of AIDS and HIV infection have become clearer and its costs to individuals and society more widely understood. Today we live in a situation where there is widespread understanding of the nature of AIDS and its mode of transmission; where some of the early fear and loathing has perhaps diminished; but where prejudice and discrimination against people with AIDS and HIV is widespread; where the disease has been defined as a major public issue deserving of public funding, though still not to the degree necessary; and where the very term AIDS still carries with it a symbolic weight it should not have to bear.

Issues

I now want to turn to a number of key issues raised by this attempt at a typology of the AIDS crisis so far, because these provide the agenda which must be addressed if we want to move beyond crisis management towards a more rational and long term strategy. As Cindy Patton has remarked:

> . . . To those outside AIDS organizing, AIDS continues to be viewed primarily as a single issue. To those inside, the range and complexity of issues tapped seems almost impossible to combat . . . (Patton, 1985)

It is the complexity of these issues which most needs discussion because it will help us grasp why AIDS carries such a burden of meaning. I want to isolate a number of critical themes which illustrate this complexity.

Historical and Social Science Issues

The key problem here is: why did *this* disease, at this particular time, become the symbolic carrier of such a weight of meaning. Other new diseases have emerged in the recent past — Legionnaire's Disease is the best known — and there have been epidemics of others. Some, such as genital herpes and hepatitis B, have caused major bouts of anxiety and much social philosophizing, in ways that prefigure the reaction to AIDS. But it was AIDS that became the disease of the 1980s, and it was AIDS that came to public consciousness as the twentieth-century plague.

One of the most important factors behind this was the association of AIDS with marginal populations. As a disease that appeared to affect disproportionately black people and gay men, anxiety about AIDS was thereby able to draw on pre-existing tensions concerning race and sexual diversity, ones which were already coming to the fore in the early 1980s in the contemporary political discourse of the New Right (Hammonds, 1987). But this only pushes the question a little way back. These factors themselves clearly relate to wider anxieties. At the heart of these, I would argue, are deeply rooted fears about the unprecedented rate of change in sexual behaviour and social mores in the past two generations.

It is now quite well established that sexuality has been at the heart of public discourse since at least the early nineteenth century as a barometer of social anxiety and a conductor of social tensions. Sexuality has become both central to personal identity and a key element in social policy (Foucault, 1979).

The response to AIDS was able to draw on a variety of beliefs and concepts which often reach back into the mists of time, or at least the sexual debates of the last century. The definition of AIDS as a medico-moral problem echoes the debates in the 1830s and 1840s in England about the environmental factors associated with the spread of cholera and typhoid (Mort, 1987). The categorization of gay men as a risk category replays the definition of prostitutes as the reservoir of venereal disease in the mid-nineteenth century. Even the suggestion that those at risk should be segregated and quarantined has a precedent in the Contagious Diseases Acts of the 1860s which sought compulsorily to test women suspected of being prostitutes in various English garrison towns (Weeks, 1989). There is little new, it seems, in the field of sexual regulation.

But what is new, however, is the fluidity of sexual identities and the emergence of new sexual communities since the 1960s. These have provided opportunities for many, but anxiety for others whose own sense of self, and perception of the normal order of things, has been severely threatened by the speed of social change. Such change has provided a fertile recruitment ground for the moral politics of the New Right and has helped to create those constituencies most frightened by the emergence of AIDS (Weeks, 1985). For such people, AIDS comes to represent all the changes that have occurred over recent decades, as well as their fearful consequences. Culturally, the ground for the social reaction to AIDS was prepared before any one noticed the range of illnesses afflicting gay men and others. In a sense therefore there was already an immanent problem awaiting a symbolic resolution. To this extent, AIDS was a crisis waiting to happen.

Political Issues

AIDS is a cultural phenomenon, but in an age when culture and politics are more inextricably mingled than ever before, and when the politicization of everyday life continuously expands, it is inevitable that it should also become a political issue. AIDS first appeared in a period of profound political re-formation in most Western countries, represented most clearly by the rise of the New Right inflected administrations of Reagan in the USA and Thatcher in Britain.

The significance of this political shift for AIDS was two-fold. First, these governments were ideologically committed to cutting government expenditure at a time when the emergence of a major health crisis clearly demanded a substantial increase in governmental spending on health services. After 1985, resources were indeed put into AIDS support services and AIDS-related research, but more often than not the sums involved were much less than was demanded by those in the front line. They were also often provided as part of a redistribution of resources within an already determined budget (Shilts, 1988; Small, 1988).

A clear example of this occurred in March 1988 when the British government decided it could allocate no extra cash to implement a series of measures designed to stop the spread of HIV infection through injecting drug use despite the advice received from its own statutory body, the Advisory Council on Misuse of Drugs. A newspaper report summarized the government's position thus:

> The government acknowledges the importance of the preventative measures which have been recommended by the council but has only agreed to continue a £1m allocation first made a year ago. New services need to be created for addicts and existing services expanded, the Department of Health says in a circular to health authorities and local authorities, but no additional means will be provided to achieve these aims. (*The Independent*, 30 March 1988)

Governments always have to prioritize expenditure decisions, and no-one could realistically expect that in a world of finite resources all that is demanded can be readily provided. But clearly also decisions about AIDS funding have been shaped by wider political considerations. In the case just cited, it was politically difficult for a government committed to a moral crusade against drugs to simultaneously fund syringe exchange schemes — an action likely to be seen by its more avid supporters as condoning drug abuse. From the beginning of the crisis, there has therefore been an ultimately irresolvable contradiction between the needs of people with AIDS and the political imperatives of New Right regimes.

This brings me to the second political factor relevant to AIDS, the importance of symbolic issues in New Right politics in the 1980s. In both the USA and Britain, high priority has been given to restoring national pride and economic strength. This has produced material effects (strengthened defence, a more nationalistic foreign policy, economic well-being), but also a number of less tangible outcomes: a desire to 'walk tall' in the world, a desire to restore old values and so on.

At the centre of New Right discourse has been a symbolic crusade against what were seen as the moral excesses of the 1960s and 1970s, what in Britain has been called 'permissiveness', and an effort to reaffirm traditional family and sexual values. In practical terms, the effects have been limited. President Reagan found it virtually impossible to carry through any of his family policy, and Mrs Thatcher's direct ventures into moral politics were on the whole (with some important exceptions) rhetorical rather than legislative. But New Right propagandists have been more successful in setting the terms of the debate on sexuality, and AIDS has provided a convenient marker for their case.

Thus within New Right rhetoric we can find many examples of explicit links being made between permissiveness and AIDS. To quote one recent example from a former government minister, Sir Rhodes Boyson:

> . . . It is wrong biblically, is homosexuality. It is unnatural. AIDS is, to me, a part of the fruits of the permissive society. The regular one-man, one-woman marriage would not put us at risk with this in any way . . . (*The Guardian*, 1 May 1988)

Arguments such as this help create an environment in which it becomes permissable for people to be openly hostile towards non-traditional sexual life-styles. The effects of this may be incalculable. It has been argued (Shilts, 1988) that in fact the anti-gay backlash stimulated by AIDS has been much exaggerated, and certainly there has as yet been no wholesale abrogation of gay rights in the wake of AIDS. On the other hand, there are signs of a substantial drop of support for lesbian and gay rights in Britain. An opinion poll conducted for London Weekend Television in January 1988 showed that support for the legalization of homosexual relations had dropped from 61 per cent in 1985 to 48 per cent in 1988, with over half of those polled believing that homosexuality itself was 'unnatural' (Harris Research Centre for LWT's *Weekend World*, 24 January 1988). It is difficult to find any other reason for this shift, in a climate that still remained relatively liberal on sexual matters, except for anxiety over AIDS.

Similarly, there were many factors behind the Thatcher government's introduction of measures to limit the 'promotion' of homosexuality by local authorities via Section 28 of the 1988 Local Government Act, not least the wish to wrong-foot the opposition Labour Party over its ambivalent support for gay rights. On the other hand, it is at least open to question whether the government would have intervened here were it not for the climate generated by AIDS. The introduction of Section 28 coincided with a new readiness in the tabloid (and government supporting) press to use explicit terms of abuse against lesbians and gay men, and at least part of the rationale for this new statutory limitations on gay rights suggested that they were a political response to a changing political climate on homosexuality — a climate increasingly receptive to, as well as shaped by, a wider moral-political agenda (Weeks, 1989).

It would be wrong, however, to believe that this political agenda has been easily accepted, or uncontested. One of the interesting features of the political response to AIDS has been the divisions it has revealed within the dominant political movements and agencies of government. In recent years both America and Britain have witnessed sharp, if often covert, conflicts within government about how to respond to AIDS: conflicts of priorities and of interest between politicians and civil servants, medical and scientific advisors and pressure groups (Shilts, 1988; Weeks, 1988). As a sensitive political issue, not susceptible to easy solution, AIDS has therefore provided important insights into the complexities of policy formation in pluralist societies.

Social Policy/Social Welfare Issues

These complexities help explain the difficulties associated with the development of a coherent social policy towards AIDS. In many Western countries, AIDS has erupted in a period when the Welfare State policies forged as part of the post-war social settlement have reached a period of acute crisis. Partly this is a consequence of the fiscal crisis of Welfarism, as most Western countries have found it impossible, first politically, and then ideologically, to increase expenditure on welfare services to the degree necessary to sustain their quality. This has led inevitably to the search for new policies of selectivity, targetting and privatization in order to reduce expenditure. AIDS, on the other hand, clearly demands more resources and by implication a coordinated national, and international, strategy (an issue explored more fully in Frankenberg's chapter in this volume).

There are interesting tensions at play here, for the challenge to Welfarism in the 1960s and 1970s came as much from the New Left as the New Right, though the rationale and logic were different in each case. Both however were concerned to redefine what might be an appropriate balance of public obligations and private rights.

Put at its crudest, the New Right has been essentially concerned with as far as possible diminishing the role of the state in the provision of social care, and encouraging the devolution of this responsibility to the 'private sphere'. This logically implies reliance on those community support networks that already exist, many of which have their origins within the lesbian and gay communities. This of course conflicts with a different ideological strand in the New right agenda, that which is familialist and anti-gay. In fact, as I have argued elsewhere, there has always been an uneasy contradiction in the New Right social agenda between the economic liberal and the social authoritarian (Weeks, 1985). The latter strand comes to the fore in proposals for the segregation of people with AIDS, for compulsory testing, and for stringent immigration control. But such proposals scarcely augur well for trust in the community and the diminution of state involvement that the other component of this agenda advocates.

The New Left position, on the other hand, is not without equivalent contradictions. A progressive approach to social policy assumes two things: that it is possible to develop a spirit of altruism, social responsibility and solidarity in the population at large; and that this will be accompanied by the democratization and social accountability of the services provided by and for the community and its constituent parts. With regard to AIDS, this has led to some problems *within* self-help groupings about the proper relationship they should have with the local and national state; and *between* self-help organizations and the state.

This situation is complicated by questions of whether self-help organizations should act as pressure groups or campaigning organizations for better governmental involvement in the fight against AIDS, or the vehicles for the delivery of services (Whitehead, 1988), which in turn raises fundamental issues about both accountability and professionalization. Cindy Patton has raised these problems in her attack on what she calls the 'AIDS industry'. She argues that in the US there was a major shift in the fight against AIDS between mid-1985 and mid-1986 away from gay movement inspired organizational forms and resistance to a hostile government and the medical establishment, and towards a mode of professionalization which separated the new industry from its original roots. The politics of gay liberation lost out to what Patton calls the 'new altruism', an outcome complicit with the privatizing zeal of the New Right (Patton, 1988).

Often, therefore, the self-help organizations become service agencies, increasingly reliant on state funding. At the same time, more militant groupings emerge to reaffirm the original radicalism. The problem with this position is that it is in danger of ignoring the fact that AIDS is much more than a gay issue, and that many of the groups worst affected by AIDS do not have the organizational traditions to be able to sustain a fight against AIDS without the support of other, better organized groups.

These debates raise a number of fundamental issues about social policy: about the balance between the needs of individuals and communities of choice, about the conflict between the demands of governments for appropriate accountability and standards of professionalism, and the fear of politicians that they may be seen to be acting on behalf of unpopular special interests. A few examples do exist of a close relationship between community groups and other voluntary and government agencies serving the needs of individuals and groups at risk (see Sheffield AIDS Education Project, 1987; Homans and Aggleton, 1988). It is important to recognise though that these represent attempts to work out new ways of relating need to service provision under the pressure of a health crisis. They are thus *new* models for social policy rather than traditional ones.

Medico-Moral Issues

All these debates are framed by what we can term 'medico-moral' issues. It has long been clear that medicine is far from being the neutral force that its own history would generally have us believe. Medicine is deeply involved in the relations of power — and hence the morals — of the culture in which it is embedded. One has only to think of the different medical cultures in the US and Britain, the first rooted in a private enterprise culture where medical services are sold, and the second in a welfarist and altruistic tradition where medicine is a service to be provided, to realize the profoundly different outcomes that are likely to emerge. To take a simple example, which had a bearing on the early history of the AIDS crisis: blood is still often sold in the USA; in Britain it is contributed voluntarily, as part of the 'gift relationship' which underpinned the formation of the National Health Service. This difference can have profound effects (Weeks, 1985).

Medicine is an essential element in the fight against AIDS, but it has also been a constituent agent in the formation of 'AIDS' as a social issue. The medical profession, for example, played a major role in defining homosexuality as a disease during the course of the past century (Weeks, 1977). The easy slippage that took place in the early stages of the present health crisis which encouraged AIDS to be seen as a disease of diseased people owed a great deal to that tradition, challenged during the years of gay liberation, but continuing nevertheless as an unconscious element in medical discourse. A recent example of this in Britain is provided by a group of 'Christian doctors' who proposed to halt the epidemic by segregating and isolating tens of thousands of people carrying the virus (Collier, 1987).

These are minority views, yet this history has powerfully structured the relations between the communities most affected by AIDS and the medical profession itself. There can be no doubt that the response of many gay activists to AIDS in the early years of the crisis was shaped by a deeply rooted fear of the 're-medicalization' of homosexuality. More recently, Silverman (in this book) has compared the 'culturally-shared moral forms' of the people with HIV that he observed in a medical situation to the clinical approach of the doctors. Part of this is a necessary balance; part of it reflects a cultural divide.

At the same time, as Silverman goes on to argue, the publicity given to HIV infection and AIDS, and the structures of the community most affected by AIDS in the West, mean that patients are more knowledgeable than usual about official as opposed to folk or lay health knowledge (see Fitzpatrick, Boulton and Hart in this volume). In turn, many of the medical personnel involved in caring for people with AIDS are themselves from the community itself. This makes for major challenges to the traditional clientillistic relationship between doctor and patient. Here too, *new* models of social interaction and care may emerge in response to the health crisis.

International Issues

So far, I have concentrated on a limited range of national and Western responses. But AIDS is of course an international crisis. This poses questions about the necessity, and difficulty, of international cooperation to deal with AIDS in a world riven by political, economic and ideological divisions. It is surely significant that even as countries come together to find ways of cooperating, the way in which AIDS is understood is highly culturally specific. Western countries debate whether students or long-term residents from Third World countries should be compulsorily tested. At the same time, others from the developing world bitterly resent suggestions that the disease originated and spread from Africa and see this as a typical piece of neo-colonial and racist propaganda (Chirimuuta and Chirimuuta, 1987; Mercer, 1988).

At an international meeting of health ministers early in 1988, the Princess Royal suggested that AIDS was an 'own goal' for mankind (*The Guardian*, 27 January 1988), as if blame could be collectively attributed to particular groups of people. Suggestions like these inevitably lead to the assumption that there are 'innocent' and 'guilty' victims of the disease (Watney, 1988). Apart from the ethics of so differentiating between those infected, there is an underlying philosophical dilemma; whom you regard as innocent and whom guilty is ultimately a matter of where you live and whom you stand with. The truth is that while AIDS as a syndrome of diseases has common features in all parts of the world, the social meanings it gives rise to can be profoundly different. If this is the case, it has implications for the ways in which AIDS is likely to be coped with in each culture. In the years ahead we will therefore need to adjust the treatment of AIDS to local customs and traditions, and to specific social and ethical values.

Nevertheless, AIDS is potentially a crisis of global proportions. It has implications for population growth and for the structure of family and sexual relations. It has troubling financial and economic consequences for a world economy already dangerously unbalanced, and incapable of finding commonly agreed solutions to already identified problems, let alone new, and politically fraught, health issues. Above all, it pinpoints both the challenge, and hazardous nature, of international cooperation.

Personal and Community Issues

Finally, I want to return to the personal, to people with HIV infection and/or AIDS, and to the communities to which they belong. James Baldwin once remarked, 'That isolation and death are certain and universal clarifies our responsibility' (Baldwin, 1986). As members of the community most affected, lesbians and gay men have had to learn this lesson very rapidly. In a world where the dying have conventionally 'been removed so hygienically behind the scenes of social life' (Elias, 1985), people have suddenly needed to come to terms with illness, bereavement and loss on a massive scale. Yet the evidence is overwhelming that far from buckling under the strain, ties of community in the lesbian and gay world have been strengthened during these years. As Shilts remarks, at the end of a book which is otherwise partisan and critical of many aspects of gay life during the

1980s, '. . . there was a new community emerging . . . of people who had learned to take responsibility for themselves and for each other' (Shilts, 1988). There is a paradox here worth pondering on: suffering and bereavement appear to bring people together in a way that health and prosperity do not.

Conclusion

It will not have escaped anyone's attention that none of the issues discussed above are peculiar to AIDS. This echoes my conviction that the only way to understand the political and ethical implications of AIDS is to see it in a wider social context: of rapid social change and the anxieties attendant upon this, especially those changes which have affected sexual behaviour and values, race and social non-conformity; of political and moral struggles in which old certainties have collapsed and new and competing ones emerged; of new personal identities, many of them now fashioned in the furnace of personal suffering.

I began by describing three phases within the AIDS crisis so far, and suggested that we are currently living through a period of crisis management. This by definition means that we are addressing symptoms rather than fundamental causes. The subsequent discussion of key issues suggests that latent in the current situation is a more developed and rational response based on a realistic assessment of risk, a balanced understanding of the nature of AIDS and HIV infection, an awareness of the resources needed to deal with this, and the political and moral will necessary to find and use those resources. The challenge to society and governments in the next few years lies in harnessing this potential in order to move toward a more rational and progressive solution.

In many ways AIDS is like many other illnesses which devastate individual lives. What is remarkable about AIDS, however, is not simply its virulence, but the weight of symbolic meaning that it carries. Because of this, it throws into sharp focus the murkier preoccupations of our age. It carries a burden which those who experience it most personally should not have to bear. Perhaps the real signal that a new period is upon us will come when AIDS does become just another disease demanding the same care, attention and social resources as any other.

References

AGGLETON, P. and HOMANS, H. (Eds.) (1988) *Social Aspects of AIDS*, Lewes, Falmer Press.
ALCORN, K. (1988) 'Illness, metaphor and AIDS', in AGGLETON, P. and HOMANS, H. (Eds.) *Social Aspects of AIDS*, Lewes, Falmer Press.
BALDWIN, J. (1986) *Evidence of Things Not Seen*, London, Michael Joseph.
BERKOWITZ, R. and CALLEN, M. (1983) *How to Have Sex in an Epidemic*, New York, News from the Front.
CHIRIMUUTA, R. and CHIRIMUUTA, R. (1987) *AIDS, Africa and Racism*, available from R. Chirimuuta, Bretby House, Stanhope, Bretby, Burton-on-Trent, DE15 OPT.
COLLIER, C. (1987) *The Twentieth Century Plague*, London, Lion.
ELIAS, N. (1985) *The Loneliness of the Dying*, Oxford, Basil Blackwell.
FOUCAULT, M. (1979) *The History of Sexuality, Volume 1, An Introduction*, London, Allen Lane.
HAMMONDS, E. (1987) 'Race, sex, AIDS: The construction of the other', *Radical America* 20, 6.
HOMANS, H. and AGGLETON, P. (1988) 'Health education, HIV infection and AIDS', in AGGLETON, P. and HOMANS, H. (Eds.) *Social Aspects of AIDS*, Lewes, Falmer Press.
McKIE, R. (1986) *Panic, The Story of AIDS*, London, Thorsons.
MERCER, K. (1988) 'AIDS, racism and homophobia', *New Society*, 5 February.
MORT, F. (1987) *Dangerous Sexualities*, London, Routledge and Kegan Paul.
PADGUG, R. (1986) 'AIDS in historical perspective', paper presented at the American Historical Association, 28 December.
PATTON, C. (1985) *Sex and Germs. The Politics of AIDS*, Boston, MA, South End Press.
PATTON, C. (1988) 'The AIDS Industry: Construction of victims, volunteers and experts', paper presented at AIDS: The Cultural Agenda Conference, Institute of Contemporary Arts, London, 5–6 March.
SHEFFIELD AIDS EDUCATION PROJECT (1988) *Interim Report, May–October 1987*, Sheffield, Sheffield City Polytechnic.
SHILTS, R. (1988) *And the Band Played On. Politics, People and the AIDS Epidemic*, Harmondsworth, Penguin Books.
SMALL, N. (1988) 'AIDS and social policy', *Critical Social Policy*, 21, pp 9–29.
SONTAG, S. (1983) *Illness as Metaphor*, Harmondsworth, Penguin Books.
SPENCE, C. (1986) *AIDS, Time to Reclaim our Power*, London, Lifestory.
TATCHELL, P. (1986) *AIDS, A Guide to Survival*, London, Gay Men's Press.
TREICHLER, P. (1987) 'AIDS, homophobia and biomedical discourse: An epidemic of signification', *Cultural Studies*, 1, 3.
WATNEY, S. (1987) *Policing Desire*, London, Comedia/Methuen.
WATNEY, S. (1988) 'AIDS, "Moral Panic Theory" and homophobia', in AGGLETON, P. and HOMANS, H. (Eds.) *Social Aspects of AIDS*, Lewes, Falmer Press.
WEEKS, J. (1977) *Coming Out*, London, Quartet Books.
WEEKS, J. (1985) *Sexuality and its Discontents*, London, Routledge and Kegan Paul.
WEEKS, J. (1986) *Sexuality*, London, Tavistock.
WEEKS, J. (1989) *Sex, Politics and Society* (2nd edn), Harlow, Longman.
WEEKS, J. (1988) 'Love in a cold climate' in AGGLETON, P. and HOMANS, H.

(Eds.) *Social Aspects of AIDS*, Lewes, Falmer Press.
WELLINGS, K. (1988) 'Perceptions of risk — Media treatment of AIDS' in AGGLETON, P. AND HOMANS, H. (Eds.) *Social Aspects of AIDS*, Lewes, Falmer Press.
WHITEHEAD, T. (1988) Paper presented at AIDS: The Cultural Agenda Conference, Institute of Contemporary Arts, London, 5–6 March.

2
One Epidemic or Three? Cultural, Social and Historical Aspects of the AIDS Pandemic

Ronald Frankenberg

From the earliest attempts to control epidemics in the Italian City States (often even then in the interests of ruling families and groups and the commerce and interstate trade they controlled), there has been a tension between the refusal of disease to recognize local, political and social boundaries and the desires of men and women to pursue local or group interests. This tension has had a number of consequences. On the one hand, it probably led to the modern profession of spying, with Florentine health spies looking for signs of plague in Genoa. On the other, it has given rise to unparalleled co-operation, communication and mutual assistance as was the case in the seventeenth century when epidemic disease threatened to cross class and state boundaries (Cipolla, 1981).

Since the Second World War and the establishment of the United Nations and allied agencies such as UNESCO, FAO, and WHO, a chimera of international co-operation with respect to health issues has hovered ahead just out of reach of world leaders and those whom they claim to represent. Amongst these agencies, WHO has claimed important successes such as the elimination of smallpox, and has produced policy plans like the Alma Ata Declaration of 'Health for all by the year 2000', later renamed *Primary Health Care for All.* It has more or less consistently advocated a view of health that transcends curative medicine and embraced one that was at once socially and internationally-based but aimed at the individual. Nevertheless its ideas and activities tend to have reached only a medical and political elite in each member country, and the priorities of ministers and top civil servants at World Health Assemblies have often seemed to be (in contrast to resolutions passed and policies adopted) more in the interests of metropolitan exporters of drugs and technology than in those of the world's sufferers (Frankenberg and Leeson, 1974; Doyal, 1979; King, 1966).[1] This situation is complicated by the fact that high technology developments within curative medicine may well be in the interests of developing countries' ruling classes whose disease patterns may well be closer to those in developed countries than to those of their own majority urban or rural poor.

The Challenge of AIDS

Not for the first time in the field of public health, has a syndrome defined as sexually transmitted produced a qualitative change in the institutions devoted to its control (Brandt 1985; Austoker, 1987). The January 1988 London World Summit of Ministers of Health on Programmes for AIDS Prevention, sponsored jointly by WHO and the British government, attracted representatives from more countries than any previous international health meeting. It produced and unanimously approved the *London Declaration on AIDS Prevention* which emphasizes the role of health education and information in the prevention of HIV infection. According to the declaration, health education in this field 'should take full account of social and cultural patterns, different lifestyles, and human and spiritual values'. Future prevention programmes should 'protect human rights and human dignity' and 'discrimination against, and stigmatization of HIV infected people and people with AIDS undermine public health and should be avoided'.

This kind of statement is important because it establishes a moral framework, against which the actions of individual countries and states can be judged. It further provides an organizing focus for national and local struggle against broader patterns of political, racial, gender, sexual and economic discrimination. A combination of short-term geographical accident, long-term historical development, and a (hubristic?) conviction that central government can control all problems has paradoxically led a number of Socialist governments from Cuba to China by way of India and the Soviet Union to adopt their own (and in my view oppressive) policies which currently deviate from the spirit, if not the letter, of the WHO recommendations. I find it hopeful that in the long run it is these countries which have both the greatest ideological commitment and the most to gain from international co-operation.

The Three Epidemics and the Three Regional Patterns

The *London Declaration on AIDS Prevention* should, however, be seen within two rather different contexts. These were referred to by Jonathan Mann, Director of WHO's AIDS programme in his opening speech to the summit. They are the threefold differential epidemiology of HIV infection in different regions of the world, and, the three separate (but related) epidemics — of HIV infection, AIDS and social reaction to the syndrome (Mann, 1986).

AIDS itself is not a disease in the strict biomedical sense but a syndrome, a complex of symptoms and diseases which some, if not all of those infected by the Human Immunodeficiency Virus(es) (HIV) are no longer able to resist. It is not the only and possibly, in the long run, not the dominant symptom of HIV infection, which is already known to cause neurological disorder even in some people whose immune system is as yet unaffected (Wells, 1988). There is as yet no cure for nor a vaccine against HIV infection in sight, and the most optimistic predictions suggest that at least ten years will be needed before we see either. In a situation where between five and ten million people worldwide may already be infected, a biomedical remedy will clearly come too late to avert catastrophe (Mann, 1986). Prevention is not merely better than cure, it *is* the cure as epidemiologists always argue, for all three epidemics — those of HIV infection, AIDS and social reaction to the syndrome.

It cannot be emphasized too strongly that the problems raised by AIDS are international. Some of the reasons why HIV infection poses an international problem are medico-technical. The long latency period before the effects of the virus are manifest, the speed of modern travel, the impossibility of global quarantine even if this were desirable, the virus's lack of a class, race or wealth consciousness, the simultaneously imperative and infinitely diverse nature of overt and concealed sexual desire and practice — all of these factors combine to make international co-operation a necessity even for those ruling groups most self-righteously determined to go it alone. This does not, of course, mean that the kinds of co-operation which should take place are self-evident, or even that its effects will necessarily be beneficial for all. Nevertheless, part of the global impact of AIDS may be to produce what WHO has long sought for, not only a world united against disease, but a commitment to health promotion and prevention as the main means by which to bring this about. As Hafdan Mahler, Director of WHO, has said, what we once thought possible from theoretical premises we now know to be true. It is possible to check the spread of disease by health promotion at societal or communal levels. This offers new and exciting potentials for what might be called a participatory social epidemiology: a conventional epidemiology enriched and transformed by social science insights and public concern and involvement.

Regional Patterns 1: USA, the Industrial West, Australasia and Latin America

In some ways it is fortunate that AIDS was first identified in the United States, a country which, whatever the deficiencies of the medical care available to the less than wealthy, has a public health infrastructure which makes it possible to identify with speed a new set of health disorders, along with their causative mechanisms. Given the political will, a country like the United States has the financial means by which to cope with new epidemics. Had HIV infection remained prevalent only in underdeveloped or less prosperous countries, its presence might not have been recognized so quickly, and interventions against it might have come that much later. Even, or perhaps especially, in the United States, a thoroughgoing understanding of the syndrome was delayed by a clash between the institutional cultures and the derived economic priorities of two government agencies: the National Institutes for Health in Bethesda and the Centers for Disease Control in Atlanta, Georgia. The former argued initially that the latter's apparent discovery of a 'virus transmissible cancer' was simply another ploy by which to advance its economic interests. Eventually however, the two institutions were constrained to relate to one another in new and more constructive ways (Shilts, 1988).

Here in Britain, the advent of AIDS encouraged the government to give health education a more central position in the hierarchy of Health Service administration. In 1987, the semi-independent Health Education Council (HEC) became the Health Education Authority (HEA), an organization like other regional health authorities answerable to, but also with direct access to, the Secretary of State. The overt argument for this reorganization focused on the benefits that might accrue from more effective liaison to control HIV infection: the latent agenda however was one of central control by which to alleviate the embarrassment of the old HEC's attack on the tobacco, alcohol and food additive industries.

The advent of AIDS as a social phenomenon (Plummer, 1988) has therefore added new impetus to the need to understand 'How institutions think' (Douglas, 1987; Burns and Stalker, 1961). It also encourages a critical examination of the culture of the institutions in which we are embedded — be this medical, academic, gay or straight, or a combination of some or all of these. For AIDS emerged not only from San Francisco but from members of its gay community who, with needle-sharing injecting drug users and the recipients of infected blood and blood products, have borne the brunt of the HIV and AIDS epidemics as well as the epidemic of bigoted social reaction that has followed these.

This group of gay men included some who were rich and many who were well organized, culturally self-conscious as group members, and politically experienced in fighting unpopularity and overt hostility. The North American gay community had values and a style of organization which, like the other institutions already mentioned, constrained if they did not determine the actual, fantasized and self-reported behaviour of those within it. For some time prior to AIDS, out-of-the closet gay male activists had translated their desires into reality, constructing new identities and new sub-cultures within American society. They succeeded in doing this helped by a hard-won solidarity, encouraged by compassion and concern, and hindered but challenged by the often violently aggressive and viciously alienating straight world. What AIDS brought about, therefore, was in a very real sense only secondarily a change of *individual* behaviour. First and foremost, the members of an already relatively coherent *group* collectively chose to change one aspect of their culture, without abandoning that culture in its entirety. Gay sex gave way not to no sex or to a 'backsliding' repentance, but to safer sex and perhaps a deepening of relationships.

Unfortunately not all gay men in Western countries were as well placed to respond, although self-help organizations in Britain like the Terrence Higgins Trust and Body Positive have made great progress in their work, gaining as they did so somewhat grudging government support and cooperation. Many non-gays, however, have not been disposed to listen or to learn from people who at best they saw as being other than themselves, and who at worst were feared and hated for the challenge they seemed to pose to the accepted social order, the family and their own hardly (in both senses) suppressed temptations and desires.

In the last two centuries, the rich had painfully to learn that cholera and other diseases made no distinction between the deserving and the undeserving poor, still less did they differentiate between both of these groups and the rich themselves. When, because of a tendency to associate HIV's modes of transmission with 'risk groups' rather than the more epidemiologically useful 'risk behaviours', injecting drug users were added to gays, the wish to see AIDS as a problem of the other, the non-respectable, and the out-of-control, was intensified. Ironically, since in 'normal' times sufferers from genetic disorders often feel (and are) themselves stigmatized, this process was further reinforced by the ideology of the 'innocent victim', the haemophiliac infected by contaminated blood products and the baby with HIV infection.

From the point of view of controlling its spread, HIV infection amongst injecting drug users, (whether stigmatized as addicts or not) and amongst prisoners, (whether through injecting drug use or through anal intercourse), is just as worthy of attention as that in those apparently passively infected via blood transfusions or more legitimate forms of sexual activity. This may well require an overt recognition that such 'deviant' activities exist and a change in the attitude of institutions towards them. Since, unfortunately, virtue is seldom perceived as its own reward, those who see themselves as having nobly resisted such 'deviations' may need in the future to be persuaded where their real interests lie.

Regional Patterns 2: East, Central and Southern Africa, the Caribbean

The reaction to the discovery of AIDS and HIV infection amongst gay men and injecting drug users in the industrialized West was, as I have already suggested, at best, one of distanced but reproving pity. As the Princess Royal put it early in 1988 (more in sorrow than in anger), 'Mankind has scored an own goal against itself'. At worst, there have been theologically perverse (at least by New Testament standards) responses amongst members of the Moral Majority in the United States and amongst some Chief Constables and Rabbis in Britain which suggest that HIV infection and AIDS are the consequence of divine anger and retribution.

Similarly, social reaction to the discovery of widespread HIV infection amongst heterosexuals in parts of Africa only narrowly avoided the catastrophic. Western ignorance about the regional variability of HIV infection within the vast continent of Africa, alongside stereotypes of African promiscuity, led to hasty suggestions in Britain that still greater immigration and travel control over black Africans were needed. By way of contrast, few have suggested the need for stricter immigration control over white (and often rich) US citizens from areas where the incidence of HIV infection is high. This kind of reaction led some African states initially to deny that such a problem existed at all. Only careful diplomacy by WHO and the good sense of African politicians such as President Kaunda, who spoke movingly of the death of his own son, saved the situation. There still remain some, however, who deny the existence of an AIDS epidemic in Africa or who contend that African AIDS is somehow different from that seen in the West (see Chirimuuta and Chirimuuta, 1987). Whilst it is undoubtedly true that some journalists and right wing politicians were ready and indeed happy to jump to the conclusion that HIV originated in Africa, using this as yet another excuse whereby to exclude the racial 'other', in some urban areas of South Central Africa up to 25 per cent of the population between 20–40 years old may be HIV positive, and in others beween 5–15 per cent of pregnant mothers tested are known to be so.

The reasons for this high prevalence are as yet unclear although synergism between HIV and syphilis, genital lesions, malnutrition aflatoxins and other effects of poverty have all been suggested. But what is clear are the staggering implications of such figures. In some countries, the elite, who live in towns and on whom further development and national economy recovery may depend may be more than decimated. Thus productive and skilled workers and educators may be rendered ineffective, and a whole generation made virtually unable to reproduce itself. Orphans and the elderly may be left without support, and past achievement in the field of health care made impossible to maintain.

There are potential dangers also in some of the poorer areas of Southern Europe, in parts of Latin America and in Asia. Compulsory HIV testing and what seem to be punitively harsh 'medical' measures have been reported from some Latin American countries and from Cuba. In addition to being discriminatory, particularly in relation to classical 'others' such as foreigners, prostitute women and gay men, actions like these may well make matters worse by encouraging the concealment of infection.

Regional Patterns 3: Asia and Eastern Europe, the Pacific

In Asia, most of the Pacific, the Middle East and much of Eastern Europe, there have as yet been very few cases of AIDS, and the appearance of HIV infection is more recent in these parts of the world. The governments of many countries in these regions believe that AIDS is a disease brought from outside by sexual intercourse with foreigners or by the importation of infected blood products. However, there is now evidence of internal transmission in the usual ways, and even if countries succeed in carrying out the policies of isolation and (in some cases punitive compulsory) control to which they are committed, they will most probably not be able to halt the spread of HIV. Fortunately, as we have seen, despite the reservations expressed by their representatives attending the London Summit, these countries agreed to sign the *London Declaration* and are thus pledged to world co-operation in the long run.

The First Epidemic: Desire, Practice, Identity and Culture in the Prevention of HIV Infection

The first objective of WHO's global strategy on AIDS is to prevent further HIV infection. However, this cannot be achieved in isolation from, or with indifference towards, the development of AIDS in those already infected. Moreover, the attainment of this first goal has to be combined with a concern for the social experience of people who are, rightly or wrongly, believed to be at special risk, as well as for those who already are HIV seropositive and/or who have AIDS.

The lessons that we can draw from experience so far and especially from gay self-help in the industrialized world are manifold. First, it is clearly the case that the prevention of HIV transmission involves changes in sexual behaviour. Nevertheless, researchers and health promoters, whether in preventive medicine or in the media, must recognize for others as they do for their own lives, that sexual behaviours, especially those that are indicative of life style and identity, are socially determined; they are not merely the result of autonomous individual or dyadic choices (see Davies' chapter elsewhere in this volume). It is in specific, analysable but, in the last analysis, changeable circumstances that desires become transformed into practices, the symbolic markers of individual, cultural and social identities.

Surprisingly little is known about the specifics of individual sexual behaviour or even about the culturally approved practices within groups and sub-groups. Obviously straightforward questionnaire techniques are difficult to apply, and produce data of questionable reliability and validity. Amongst British sociologists, Coxon (1988a and 1988b) and his co-workers on *Project Sigma* have developed an ingenious self-reporting diary technique by which to begin to study the sexual behaviour of gay men.

Second it is not for the sociological observer to predict in what way the sexual behaviour of women and men of different groups and nationalities will change. In past pandemics, some of the threatened fled, some repented and some, in joyous despair, gave themselves up to riotous living. Within the general framework of WHO's global strategy, some countries' health education campaigns have argued not for fewer sexual acts, but for richer, more equal and safer personal relationships. Others have argued for tighter moral and legal control via monogamy or abstinence — 'Clean living is the only real safeguard', the mysterious public lavatory exhortation against syphilis and gonorrhoea of my own schooldays in World War Two. These last strategies may be more closely related to the social and ideological background of those who put them forward than to their effectiveness.

It is important to recognize that not only are government and media campaigns like these received, interpreted and acted upon within particular cultural framework, they are also produced within one. Nor are these cultural frameworks necessarily silky and seamless, homogeneous and devoid of contradiction. In this respect, it is useful to compare recent Danish and British health education campaigns directed at sexually active young people. The British approach so far has been based on the assumption that past patterns of behaviour should be condemned as, if not bad, at least amoral. It further operates from the assumption that decisions about risk-taking in sexual encounters are purely personal or at most dyadic. Even if the disco culture portrayed as a background to individual decision-taking is accurate, as it probably is, the wider social context of sought-for approval and avoidance of disapproval from important others, is conspicuously absent in recent British television commercials produced as part of this campaign. Such a strategy contrasts sharply with earlier health education campaigns on smoking but is similar to that of the recent Department of Health anti-heroin campaign that partially misfired by underestimating the subcultural attractions of male vulnerability. Recent Danish campaigns, on the other hand, begin by accepting and even applauding adolescent hedonistic values, and while they leave the choices about fundamental changes in sexual behaviour open to young people themselves, they show how existing practices can be modified to make them safer.

An even sharper contrast can be seen in Australia where the government campaign aimed at the general public has been based on images of fear and death, incorporating the Grim Reaper, skittle player and carver of tombstones (see Folio, 1988), but where there have also been community based initiatives developed from within Aboriginal culture, and in co-operation with local women, by the Aboriginal Community Health Worker Gracelyn Smallwood.

If, as is sometimes the case, rhetoric and reality coincide, then people with the same cultural background to those who have designed particular health education initiatives (see Wiseman's chapter in this volume) may be influenced by their content. If the message of what has to be avoided is made clear and the options open are then explained, those who are sufficiently convinced to feel themselves at risk will adapt their own socially interactive sense of identity and culture to the new situation as they perceive it. The critical issue of timing is emphasized, however, by those studies which suggest that there was a 25 per cent rate of HIV seropositivity amongst gay men in San Francisco before the first case of AIDS was reported. This emphasizes the need for steps to prevent the second and third epidemics.

Preventing the Second Epidemic: Living with Infection or Dying From It

At first sight, whether or when those with HIV infection will develop AIDS, AIDS-related complex or any other pathology or even die prematurely, appears to be a purely medical issue. However the epidemiology of a recognized disease always has a social component. This influences the way in which biological disorders as sickness are culturally performed (Frankenberg, 1986) — how they are diagnosed and by whom, what they are called and why, whether patients are hospitalized and when, whether they are treated and what for, and when the struggle for life ought to be, or is, abandoned.

Discussions about the last of these issues are particularly important. Prolongation of life may be seen as undesirable, when to carry on living is seen as too painful for the patient, for their relatives or loved ones, or for health care workers. This is not the least of the reasons why careful terminology is important in relation to all three epidemics.

An ill chosen or unconscious metaphor can be, even if it never appears on the death certificate, the cause of an unnecessary or premature death. Consciously or unconsciously, overtly or secretly, honestly or less honestly, choices and decisions are made, and social factors such as age, perceived quality of life, marital status, dependent children, responsibility for self and others, and 'willingness to fight' are taken into account.

HIV infection presents challenge and opportunity in all these areas and no doubt others as yet unthought of. The published literature suggests that the challenge has only been partly met and, significantly, to a much greater extent from within the gay community and by those directly affected rather than the institutionalized practices of medicine itself. In Britain, for example, it is useful to compare Tatchell's (1987) self-help manual *AIDS: A Guide to Survival* with the more liberal and less radical book by Miller, Weber and Green (1986) *The Management of AIDS Patients*. The latter title not only conceals the usefulness to patients of much that is in the book but also reveals institutional imperatives. A book entitled *Helping AIDS Patients to Help Themselves* would perhaps have bridged the cultures of patients and health workers.

Already in Britain the prescription of expensive drugs which may prevent the development of AIDS in those who have HIV infection and which, in some cases, slow down the processes associated with the syndrome itself has not been authorized for both sets of patients. Most frequently, these drugs have been given to those with AIDS but denied to those who are merely HIV antibody positive for reasons which may stem as much from a fear of expense as from concern about their possible side effects. How are such decisions going to be taken in poorer countries where just to administer HIV antibody tests for those believed to have been at risk would quickly exhaust available health budgets?

Death and Its Social Acceptance

We all live in the presence of death at an uncertain time in the future, but that does not mean that a diagnosis of HIV infection, or of other potentially terminal diseases, has to mean a sentence to die in the presence of life. Neither does it mean that those with HIV infection should be put quietly but firmly outside social life lest they remind others of their own mortality and sexuality.

Save in war and through accident, death and dementia in Western industrial society have in the twentieth century become the prerogative of the old. The process of dying is safely ignored by the rest of society, who dismiss it in practice if not in rhetoric, as something which happens to others, who with affection are said to have had their time, or with calculation, to have made their contribution. In less industrially developed, poor nations, death either comes early in childhood or still relatively late in life. In either of these contexts, AIDS threatens to interrupt conventional perceptions of death and dying by striking people who are in their procreative and productive prime. Moreover, it does not do this suddenly but with ample but uncertain warning. Medicine, social services and even family structures are not well organized to deal with the material, spiritual and social consequences of this kind of change. Outside the hospice and the geriatric ward and especially in the teaching hospitals of the West, doctors are trained to cure the acutely sick, and nurses to care for them whilst attempts at cure are made. Widespread compulsory testing would make this situation worse. Indeed private medicine in Britain and the US specifically rejects altogether responsibility for care without cure. Even before the advent of HIV infection, such models of care were increasingly seen as inappropriate, certainly within the under-developed countries (King, 1966), but also in advanced industrial societies within the context of chronic disease and high technology care (Strauss *et al*, 1985). Even where Primary Health Care is well developed, its practitioners find difficulty in meeting other than the most superficial needs of the chronic sick and dying (Cartwright *et al*, 1973).

Many patients with cancer and other diseases are told (or guess, from observing changes in the frequency of their outpatient attendance or in the provision of medication) that their days are numbered. But few are offered, even in the most developed societies, counselling on how to live their dying days, or specific advice on nutrition, exercise and staying fit. In many ways, they may in fact be worse off than their counterparts in countries where urban dwellers habitually return to their village of birth to end their days. Those diagnosed as HIV antibody positive may find themselves in an even worse position, since they are condemned to an uncertain future, complicated perhaps by ostracism, unemployment and financial difficulty (and in some cases mental decline). Uncertainty about prognosis is widely recognized as one of the major pains associated with many kinds of chronic disease and disability (Locker, 1983). Combined with the prospect of a not too distant death and possible guilt about sexual and moral lack of control, it can be a recipe for misery which, in the absence of support, may lead to suicide or deliberately anti-social behaviour.

The nature of AIDS as a super-vulnerability rather than as a specific disease puts those who have developed it on a roller coaster of possible ups and downs and ins and outs, both in relation to hospital and to the transition from patient to person and back again. This is just the kind of situation which even the most developed hospitals find it difficult to deal with, both in terms of patient welfare and their own economies.

The Family as an Answer?

In both highly industrialized societies and those that are less industrially developed, the traditional solution to this kind of problem has been the family in its various forms. In countries like Britain, the term community care is often used as a euphemism for family care, and the term family is in turn used to conceal the burdens placed on married women, who at the age of 50, may find themselves cooking, cleaning and mending for their husbands, their grandchildren, their remaining children, their own or their husbands' widowed mothers or less usually fathers, in addition to doing a part-time job outside the home (Phillipson, 1982). Such a pattern is already burdensome, and its effects can be seen in middle aged ill-health (even if this is relabelled menopausal problems). Can such a pattern be sustained in a situation where AIDS is widespread or where the woman herself has HIV infection or an AIDS-related condition? Other countries with different employment patterns such as migrant labour or high male unemployment will, of course, confront this kind of problem in different ways.

Since it is not only the most productive but the most procreative who are at risk of HIV infection, special problems are likely to arise for children perhaps already living on the edge of malnutrition whose parents are dead or too debilitated to provide for them. This situation is likely to arise regardless of the antibody status of the children themselves. Categorizing such children as 'innocent victims' may seem to be a useful tactic to draw attention to their specific plight, but may at the same time delay action until it is too late for their parents or families who may be seen, by implication, to be guilty.

The Restructuring of Old Institutions and the Creation of New Ones

If nations fail to check the growth in the number of people with HIV infection or to prevent the development of AIDS amongst those already infected, considerable resources will clearly be needed to provide drugs and hospital and home care. In addition, nurses, doctors, home-helps (where such exist) and other health workers will need re-education and training; and friends, neighbours, lovers, the wider family, traditional or alternative healers will be needed to provide the necessary complementary support. This may well bring about the creation of totally new social institutions, as has already happened with the advent of the buddy system and by self-help organizations such as Body Positive.

In the West, families and health workers may be reluctantly accustomed to looking after the dying old, and whilst the death of very young children is tragically commonplace in less developed countries, few societies find it easy to cope with the deaths of young women and men at the height of their physical and mental powers. Perhaps we may all learn through this disastrous necessity to create and foster institutions to support those, like the elderly, whose death and decline we may already regard, and even dismiss, as in some sense normal.

Preventing the Third Epidemic: Discrimination, Ostracism and Attacks on Civil Rights

The social ostracism of the sick or the potentially sick is not a new phenomenon — indeed, the lepers and their bells of mediaeval Europe are a cliche of community medicine courses. As a student in Britain in the late 1940s I became acutely aware of the social plight, in the period of transition from college to sanatorium, of those who were in the process of being diagnosed as having pulmonary tuberculosis. In much the same way, that I had earlier, as a child experienced the sense of uncleanness that marked the removal of a sibling to an isolation hospital, and the accompanying rituals of sulphur-burning, municipal fumigation.

If disease is a biological disturbance of the individual body which leads to social disruption within the body politic, a common human reaction is to turn it back on the biological. In the search for an answer to the question 'Why has this disease struck now?', there is often a switch from the search not just for individual guilt but for a guilty group. Risk groups thereby become guilt groups. Social and especially individual *behaviour* is hard to identify and observe, but social groups are often easier to pinpoint, particularly by their more or (usually) less relevant, visible, biological and surface characteristics. We are all familiar with this social process as it operates within various forms of racism and sexism. Thus, in Germany before the Second World War, Jews saw themselves as bearers of culture and religion, but the Nazis characterized them by their noses and lisps. In Britain today, many Afro-Caribbeans and South Asians seek to identify themselves by their respective historical and cultural heritages: racists characterize them by the colour of their skin. Women's claim to equality is based today on what they can do: this is rarely disputed. What is frequently called into question by men is what they are: biology is once more selectively translated into totality.

The boundary between biological disease and social sickness overlaps the boundary between life and death, the consciousness of human mortality and ultimate certainty and lack of social control over life at the moments of both potential conception and actual dying. HIV infection and subsequent AIDS (and perhaps even more poignantly HIV-induced dementia), lend themselves to being caught up in this social emotional symbolic maelstrom as gay men, those perceived as seropositive and persons with AIDS have already suffered on a grand scale.

This presents us, as has already been suggested, with the problem of distinguishing between those measures that are likely to be effective in reducing the prevalence of high risk behaviour and those, in which short term superficial rationality conceals deeply held prejudices and the social convenience of blaming an easily identified and unpopular group.

In the history of sexually transmitted disease, women have usually been ascribed this role, either because as mothers they have failed to educate, or as wives they have failed to satisfy (and therefore to control) what has been seen as the naturally overwhelming forces of male sexual desire. Alternatively, they may be blamed because, by practising prostitution they have at once undermined the family and the health of men, by wantonly providing the illegitimate social outlet for natural forces denied legitimate expression. Past epidemics or periods, usually of military origin, when the social consciousness of sexually transmitted diseases and especially syphilis has been high, have led to the persecution and imprisonment of prostitute women and proposals for tighter social control of all women (Brandt, 1985; McNeill, 1979). To suggest that prostitution plays the central role in the present pandemic is of course to propagate a falsehood and to divert attention from the risks present in all sexual relationships (Day, forthcoming). Furthermore, for women in whatever social context they practise their sexuality, the advent of HIV and AIDS has created a situation in which control over the use of their own bodies, already a moral imperative, has become not merely a health issue but a necessity for individual and societal survival. The feminist assertion that the personal is the political has become almost a truism. The implications of this for the social organization of the world's diverse societies are enormous and complex, and it is by no means as obvious as it seems to some that the result should be or will be a new, politically, coercively or technologically, imposed puritanism. This has already become apparent from the contradictory responses there have been to national health promotion strategies.

Much modern medical thinking is presented via quasi-military analogies which seek to exclude or kill micro-organisms which have invaded the body from outside (The Magic Bullet). It is not therefore surprising that quite ancient notions of quarantining, excluding or expelling the so-called 'carriers' of disease from society should be revived and that, in the light of this, groups deserving of such treatment should be seen in quasi-biological terms. These tendencies have been particularly evident in those countries where HIV infection is as yet rare and, they provide a potential source of international political conflict. Before such actions can be endorsed, it must first be asked whether they are likely to prevent the transmission of the biological agents associated with the first two epidemics discussed here or merely constitute and reinforce to the third of them. Since HIV does not necessarily infect the politically least powerful, there can be no guarantee that those most likely to be infected would be those most likely to be confined or expelled.

Conclusions

In this chapter I have tried to show how the three epidemics associated with HIV infection have already had profound effects on every aspect of social action and experience; with social relations at an international level, family and household relationships, the social control of supposedly deviant groups, or the control of women, both individually and collectively.

What I would want to emphasize in conclusion is that the social consequences of the present health crisis need not necessarily be entirely bad. Whilst the advent of HIV infection may present difficulties, it also creates challenges and opportunities. By rendering the evils of racism, sexual oppression and gross economic and health inequalities within and between nations not only obvious but also threatening to individual, social, national and international survival, it emphasizes the need for concerted and co-operative action at all these levels.

That in early 1988, it was possible to bring together most of the earth's nations and to arrive at a global strategy with some agreement as to its implementation, is one of the few glimmers of hope for a threatened world in which the consequences of technology have seemed so often to run ahead of the possibilities associated with their social control.

Note

1 See Robertson (1984) for a general account of how an international culture of planners can come to be more influential than a national or regional culture of need.

References

Austoker, J. (1987) 'AIDS and homosexuality in Britain: An historical perspective', paper given at the BSA Medical Sociology Conference, York.

Brandt, A. (1985) *No Magic Bullet*, New York, Oxford University Press.

Burns, T. and Stalker, G. M. (1961) *The Management of Innovation*, London, Tavistock.

Cartwright, A., Hockey, L. and Anderson, J.L. (1973) *Life Before Death*, London, Routledge and Kegan Paul.

Chirimuuta, R. and Chirimuuta, R. (1987) *AIDS, Africa and Racism*, available from R. Chirimuuta, Bretby House, Stanhope, Bretby, Burton-on-Trent, DE15 OPT.

Cipolla, C. M. (1981) *Fighting the Plague in Seventeenth Century Italy*, Madison, WI, Wisconsin University Press.

Coxon, T. (1988a) 'The numbers game — Gay lifestyles, epidemiology of AIDS and social science' in Aggleton, P. and Homans, H. (Eds.) *Social Aspects of AIDS*, Lewes, Falmer Press.

Coxon, T. (1988b) 'Something sensational: The sexual diary as a research method in the study of sexual behaviour of gay males', *Sociological Review*, 36, 2, pp 352–67.

DOUGLAS, M. (1987) *How Institutions Think*, London, Routledge and Kegan Paul.

DOYAL, L. (1979) *The Political Economy of Health*, London, Pluto Press.

FOLIO (1988) Dossier on National AIDS Campaigns, Geneva, WHO.

FRANKENBERG, R. (1986) 'Sickness as cultural performance: Drama, trajectory and pilgrimage; Root metaphors and the making social of disease', *International Journal of Health Services*, 16, 4, pp 603–26.

FRANKENBERG, R. (1988) Life: Cycle, trajectory or pilgrimage? A social production approach to marxism, metaphor and mortality', in BRYMAN, A. *et al* (Eds.) *Rethinking the Life Cycle*, London, Allen and Unwin.

FRANKENBERG, R. AND LEESON, J. (1974) 'The sociology of health dilemmas in the post colonial world: Intermediate technology and medical care in Zambia, Zaire and China' in DE KADT, E. and WILLIAMS, G. (Eds.) *Sociology and Development*, London, Tavistock.

KING, M. (1966) *Medical Care in Developing Countries*, Nairobi, Oxford University Press.

LOCKER, D. (1983) *Disability and Disadvantage*, London, Tavistock.

MCNEILL, W.H. (1979) *Plagues and Peoples*, Harmondsworth, Penguin Books.

MANN, J. (1986) 'Global AIDS: Epidemiology, impact, projections and the global strategy', address to World Summit on AIDS (1988), London, January.

MILLER, D., WEBER, J. and GREEN, J. (1986) *The Management of AIDS Patients*, London, Macmillan.

PHILLIPSON, C. (1982) *Capitalism and the Construction of Old Age*, London, Macmillan.

PLUMMER, K. (1988) 'Organizing AIDS' in AGGLETON, P. and HOMANS, H. (Eds.) *Social Aspects of AIDS*, Lewes, Falmer Press.

ROBERTSON, A. F. (1984) *People and the State: An Anthropology of Planned Development*, Cambridge, Cambridge University Press.

SHILTS, R. (1987) *And the Band Played On*, New York, St. Martins Press.

STRAUSS, A., FAGERHAUGH, S., SICZEK, B. AND WIENER, C. (1985) *Social Organization of Medical Work*, Chicago, IL, Chicago University Press.

TATCHELL, P. (1987) *AIDS: A Guide to Survival*, London, Gay Men's Press.

WELLS, N. (1988) *The AIDS Virus*, London, Office of Health Economics.

3
Undergraduates' Beliefs and Attitudes About AIDS

Stephen Clift and David Stears

In this chapter we will report on some of the findings from a study of undergraduate students' beliefs and attitudes regarding AIDS carried out in late 1986 and early 1987. The fieldwork was carried out at Christ Church College, Canterbury — a college of higher education with a strong commitment to the education and training of teachers. In October 1986 an issue of Christ Church College Students' Union newspaper appeared which carried a four-page article entitled 'Everything you've ever wanted to know about contraception but never dared to ask'. The article surveyed commonly used forms of contraception, identified their advantages and disadvantages and concluded with the following word of warning:

> Because of the large ratio of women to men at this college there's always going to be a certain amount of men (though by no means all) whose one aim is to sleep with as many women as possible. They are, of course, very good at sweet talking women into believing that they are special, when really all they want is a good bonk, then 'goodbye', no ties, no tomorrow. So beware, remember the best form of contraception is the word 'NO' — this is more effective when used at the bar, rather than in the bedroom.

What was immediately striking to us about the article, however, was the lack of any reference to AIDS. Condoms were discussed, and were said to provide 'some protection against STD', but this information was rather lost in the mass of additional information provided.

Also in October 1986, *National Student* magazine, free to all members of the National Union of Students, included a special report on 'Safer sex' and 'The new puritanism' (Taggart, 1986). Introduced on the cover as 'Safe-sex super-lovers thwart death-bug horror', the article explored the challenge of changing social attitudes towards sexuality and sex education. It recommended the use of condoms and provided advice on reducing risks of infection by practising 'safer sex'. More interesting than the article itself, however, were the letters it provoked. These were published in the following issue — all were critical and one was vitriolic in its condemnation of those individuals and groups seen to be responsible for the spread of AIDS. We quote from some of the letters it contained,

> As a first year student and a new reader I was shocked to find *National Student* replete with expletives . . . The report on safer sex was disturbing. As I know the vast majority of students are not homosexuals, the report was totally unnecessary for a student magazine.

> Here we have an article . . . openly promoting young people to lead obscure lives that could damage or even kill them (physically and mentally) . . . Are normal people going to let these pitiful people promote these disgusting antics and successfully pervert students' minds, or are we going to have the guts to oppose these fashionable idiots. . . . Surely your article should be directed at those who wish to carry out a normal, natural relationship not these 'bum bandits' who think they are doing such a marvellous job to promote students' welfare. (*National Student*, 1986)

Given indications locally of a lack of awareness among students concerning AIDS as a health issue, and given the attitudes expressed in these letters, it seemed timely to conduct research to explore students' beliefs and attitudes with respect to AIDS, and to provide students and staff with information and an opportunity to discuss the syndrome's personal and social implications.

A further stimulus to pursuing such work came from our experiences participating in a two-day workshop organized by the South East Thames Regional Health Authority on 'Facts and feelings about AIDS'. The first day of this consisted of a series of participatory and experiential exercises designed to facilitate the exploration of values, feelings and attitudes in relation to sexuality and was followed during day two with factual input on the syndrome, its epidemiology, routes of transmission and safer sex. The organization and content of the workshop served to contrast very sharply the sophistication of current scientific and medical understanding of HIV infection and AIDS, with the lack of any comparable theoretical and research input on the psychological, social and educational dimensions of AIDS. Whilst it is obviously important in a training context to explore the personal and social implications of AIDS in relation to participants' own values and experience, it is equally important to consider theoretical perspectives and research findings which can inform our thinking, feeling and action regarding the social and educational implications of AIDS.

On this basis we set about carrying out a small-scale study to explore undergraduate students' awareness, beliefs and attitudes regarding HIV infection and AIDS.

The Questionnaire

A three-part questionnaire was designed for collecting information from students. In developing and piloting this, we sought the advice of groups of undergraduate students, teachers and health professionals on in-service courses and members of the college staff. The questionnaire was constructed in three parts.[1] The first of these asked for information on sex, age, parental status and previous employment. It also assessed understanding of the acronyms AIDS and HIV. The second part consisted of fifty-six statements about HIV infection and AIDS with a 5-point response format from 'strongly agree' to 'strongly disagree'. Statements were designed to assess both beliefs and attitudes on a wide variety of issues associated with AIDS. The writing of items for section 2 was guided by the trichotomous conception of attitudes as an internally consistent set of cognitive, affective and conative components (Jaspers, 1978). Items were included which focused on what students believed to be the case regarding HIV infection and AIDS, how they felt about the issues raised and how they believed they would behave in circumstances involving people who were either HIV antibody positive or who had AIDS. Some items, however, had a bearing on two or three of these aspects and represent an amalgam of these components. Finally, the third part of the questionnaire asked for personal information about religous beliefs, political affiliation, sexual activity and sexual preference.

Data Collection

Given the focus of this study on one college population of undergraduate students, it would have been possible to sample randomly from the college roll and send out questionnaires for return. We felt, however, that there were several disadvantages with such an approach, not least the likelihood that a certain percentage of questionnaires would not be returned and that students might compare, discuss and modify their answers before returning them. Instead, we decided to administer the questionnaires during course time. This was approved by the college Principal and negotiated and agreed with course tutors.

Undergraduates at Christ Church College fall into two major groups: BEd students involved in initial teacher education and BA or BSc students following joint honours degree courses in a wide variety of subject combinations. Whilst we have surveyed the beliefs and attitudes of both of these groups of students, we will report here on the work we have carried out with the BA and BSc students. Data was collected from the two largest non-overlapping subject groups (i.e. subjects that cannot be combined in a single joint honours programme). These groups comprised educational studies and radio, film and television studies students. It was possible to collect data from almost all the first and second year students and most of the third year students. Moreover, because the numbers of women and men involved was about equal, this choice of groups allows an exploration of possible sex differences. First year students were followed up after six months to identify any areas in which their views had changed.

Questionnaires were administered to students in groups under standardized conditions. All administrators were given the same instructions to read out and students were asked to space themselves apart in order to help reduce any embarrassment which some students might have felt when completing the questionnaire. Students were assured that completed questionnaires were anonymous and would be treated as completely confidential. It was also stressed that no one should feel under any obligation to participate in the study. If necessary, the questionnaire could be left unanswered.

Data were collected first during the third week in November 1986. We were thus in a position to collect information before the UK government's television advertisement campaign and leaflet drop at the end of 1986 and before media coverage of AIDS during 'AIDS week' in February 1987. The questionnaire was readministered to first year students six months later in order to monitor changes in beliefs and attitudes about AIDS.

Anticipated Outcomes

Apart from being informed by the trichotomous conception of attitudes, the present project was not based on a formally stated theoretical model of beliefs and attitudes and their relationship with behaviour. Consequently, it was not designed to test specific predictions derived from such a model. In this sense, the project should be viewed as exploratory in character. We saw it as providing a basis on which to develop a research programme which would be theory-driven to a greater extent.

Despite the lack of a formal theoretical base, we did have a number of broad expectations about what our survey would show. These were based on issues identified in published sources on AIDS and in the media, general trends emerging from research on attitudes towards social issues and our experience of discussing AIDS with students, teachers and health professionals. Pratt (1986), for example, has suggested that reactions towards AIDS have been dominated by 'fear, ignorance and prejudice', and a distinction is commonly drawn in discussion of AIDS between knowledge of 'the facts' (as opposed to uncertainty and misunderstanding) and views about its social, religious and moral significance. We expected, therefore, to find distinctions like these reflected in the pattern of responses to sets of items relating to different issues.

More specifically, we had the following expectations. First, we anticipated that items expressing anxiety, worry and fear about contact with people with HIV infection and/or AIDS would form a consistent cluster, defined also by items relating to knowledge and awareness. Second, we expected to find a second looser cluster of items related to moralism, punitiveness and homophobia: moralism being shown by a tendency to attribute AIDS to low moral standards and 'promiscuity', punitiveness by the advocacy of strong measures to deal with infected individuals, and homophobia by the holding of negative attitudes towards gay men and their position with respect to AIDS.

Finally we felt that attitudinal responses would show relationships with sex, measures of religious belief, political affiliation, sexual activity and sexual preference. Women, non-religious and left of centre students were expected to express more liberal attitudes, as were more sexually experienced students and those defining themselves as other than 'exclusively heterosexual'.

Findings

The Sample

As can be seen from table 3.1, just over half of the sample are women, over 90 per cent were aged between 18 and 29 and over half described themselves as 'religious'. A sex difference was apparent here, with women being more likely than men to hold religious beliefs ($t = 2.12$, $p < 0.05$). In terms of politics, students in the sample were spread out across the left-right spectrum with only a small percentage identifying themselves as definitely on the right or left, and with over a fifth being either uncertain or 'non-political'. In terms of sexual experience, just under half the sample were currently involved in a relationship and half were not. Both of the variables total number of partners and number of partners during the last twelve months had a strong positive skew, with a majority of students reported between 0 and 4 sexual partners, but with frequencies dropping off as the number increased. Sex differences were also apparent on these measures with men reporting more sexual partners. For the total number (men $\bar{x} = 5.60$ and women $\bar{x} = 3.80$; $t = 1.19$; n.s.) the difference was not statistically significant although this may be accounted for by the fact that the highest figure of 100 partners was reported by a woman. For the number in the last twelve months, however, the difference in means between men and women was significant (men $\bar{x} = 2.20$, women $\bar{x} = 1.20$; $t = 2.72$, $p < 0.05$). On the measure of sexual preference, over three-quarters of the sample rated themselves exclusively heterosexual. Only four students described themselves as bisexual and none reported being either exclusively or predominantly homosexual. It is clear, therefore, that women in the sample appear to be more religious and less sexually active (on the measures reported here) than the men. Given these differences, it could be argued that men and women should be treated separately for purposes of analysis. This issue was explored further by comparing men's and women's responses on the fifty-six items contained in section 2 of the questionnaire.

Table 3.1 Sample characteristics (n = 184)

1 Sex	Male	41.8%		Female	58.2%
2 Age	18–19 yrs.	37.5%		40–49 yrs.	2.7%
	20–29 yrs.	53.3%		Not given	0.5%
	30–39 yrs.	6.0%			
3 *Religious belief*	Yes	39.2%	No 57.6%	Not given	3.3%
4 *Political position*					
Definitely on the right		4.3%	Definitely on the left		8.7%
Towards the right		19.6%	Non-political		13.0%
In the centre		19.0%	Unsure/undecided/don't know		9.2%
Towards the left		22.8%	Not given		3.3%
5 *Current sexual relationship*	Yes	46.2%;	No 47.3%	Not given	6.5%
6 *Total number of sexual partners*					
	0	14.7%		6–10	13.0%
	1	23.4%		11–15	2.7%
	2–3	19.0%		20–100	3.3%
	4–5	6.5%		Not given	17.4%
7 *Numbers of partners in last 12 months*					
	0	20.1%		6–10	4.9%
	1	41.3%		11–15	0.5%
	2–3	13.65%		Not given	15.2%
	4–5	4.3%			
8 *Sexual preference*					
	Exclusively heterosexual		77.7%		
	Predominantly heterosexual		10.9%		
	Bisexual		2.2%		
	Undecided/uncertain/don't know		1.6%		
	Not given		7.6%		

Sex Differences

Out of fifty-six items, only ten provided evidence of statistically significant differences between men and women. These are reported in table 3.2.

It is clear that the differences which do emerge are rather small and there is no evidence of polarization by sex. Both sexes agreed, for example, that instruction on avoiding infection should be given in school (item 16), but agreement with this statement was somewhat stronger among men. On the basis of these results, men appear to be slightly more concerned personally about AIDS (items 3 and 15), more likely to view physical contact with an infected person as risky (items 27 and 48), but less likely to say they would insist on a potential sexual partner taking the HIV test (item 49). In addition, men were

Table 3.2 Sex differences in individual items

	Item		Men	Women	t
3	The AIDS problem is something which I haven't given much thought to and doesn't really interest me.	x̄ s.d. n	4.00 1.04 77	4.34 0.73 107	−2.44*
15	I am personally concerned about the possibility of catching AIDS sometime in the future.	x̄ s.d. n	2.71 1.16 77	3.06 0.98 105	−2.11*
16	Instruction on how to avoid catching the AIDS virus should be given to all fifth and sixth form pupils in school.	x̄ s.d. n	1.42 0.57 77	1.64 0.72 107	−2.31*
27	I would be reluctant to sit next to someone I knew to be carrying the AIDS virus.	x̄ s.d. n	3.49 1.36 77	3.87 1.11 107	−1.99*
33	The use of the sheath during sexual intercourse should be recommended in TV advertisements as a 'safe sex' practice which reduces the risk of catching AIDS.	x̄ s.d. n	1.82 0.70 77	2.12 0.91 106	−2.55*
37	I would feel disgusted by explicit descriptions of sexual acts associated with the transmission of AIDS	x̄ s.d. n	4.33 0.80 77	4.02 0.92 107	2.41*
40	I don't feel much sympathy for anyone who catches the AIDS virus through having a number of sexual partners.	x̄ s.d. n	3.99 0.97 77	3.65 1.06 107	2.21*
48	It is dangerous to touch or kiss someone who has developed AIDS and is dying as a result.	x̄ s.d. n	3.22 1.07 76	3.57 0.92 107	−2.30*
49	Before having a sexual relationship with someone I would insist that he/she have a blood test for the AIDS virus.	x̄ s.d. n	3.84 0.89 77	3.57 0.79 107	2.16*
51	I find the following statement offensive: 'no fucking without a condom' (*National Student* Magazine, October 1986)	x̄ s.d. n	3.69 1.26 77	3.30 1.09 107	2.18*

* $p < 0.05$ (two tailed)

more in favour of education and information on AIDS (items 16 and 33), less offended by explicit accounts of sexual practices and explicit language (items 37 and 51) and more sympathetic towards cases where HIV is contracted via sexual activity (item 40). Given the small number and size of differences between men and women, we considered it reasonable for the purposes of the present investigation to regard men and women as a single group. We looked next for areas of consensus, uncertainty and divergence in responses to the questionnaire items and then explored the clustering of responses to individual items.

Beliefs and Attitudes About HIV Infection and AIDS

Table 3.3 reports results for three sets of sixteen items showing the highest levels of consensus, uncertainty and divergence. A number of items showed both uncertainty and divergence and these are separated in section 4 of the table.

For most of the items on which consensus was obtained, the level of agreement or disagreement was higher than 70 per cent, and in many cases a substantial proportion of students expressed strong agreement or disagreement. The picture which emerged is perhaps fairly predictable, and the largest group of items related to the need for public information and education. Students reported having given some thought to issues to do with AIDS, they clearly endorsed the need for public information and agreed that education in schools should provide information on 'safer sex'. Explicit descriptions of sexual activity were not regarded as disgusting, and explicit references to anal intercourse, barrier contraceptives and 'safe sex' techniques were advocated. A majority of students were in favour of supplying clean needles to injecting drug users.

A second group of items related to the likelihood of change in sexual behaviour. Most students appeared to be pessimistic about the likelihood of significant changes in patterns of sexual behaviour and contraceptive use, at least in the short term. A third group of items related to sexual activity with more than one partner. Such activity was seen as carrying a risk and someone who is HIV antibody positive and who engages in sexual activity with more than one partner was almost unanimously considered to be irresponsible. Advice on 'safe sex' was not seen as a rearguard action on the part of those wishing to defend sexual promiscuity. Finally, students clearly rejected the idea that AIDS was a form of divine intervention prompted either by the general trend towards greater sexual permissiveness in society or as a punishment for the 'sin' of homosexuality. There was also clear rejection of strongly homophobic sentiments and discriminatory action by employers against people with HIV infection.

Table 3.3 Areas of relative consensus, uncertainty and divergence in students' view on HIV/AIDS

	% Agree	% Uncertain	% Disagree
1 *Statements where there was consensus on agreement*			
23 Any one who knows they have the AIDS virus and engages in sexual activity with more than one partner is behaving irresponsibly.	98.4	1.6	0.0
6 The government's proposed TV campaign should tell people in explicit language about the ways they can catch the AIDS virus.	95.1	2.7	2.2
16 Instruction on how to avoid catching the AIDS virus should be given to all fifth and sixth form pupils in school.	95.1	3.3	1.6
28 Fifth and sixth form pupils should be taught about 'safe sex' practices, i.e. those which carry a low risk of transmitting the AIDS virus.	87.0	7.6	5.4
11 Patterns of sexual behaviour in our society will not change quickly enough to avoid further spread of AIDS	78.2	16.9	4.9
4 At present, anyone who has more than one sexual partner runs some risk of catching the AIDS virus.	75.0	15.2	9.8
33 The use of a sheath during sexual intercourse should be recommended in TV advertisements as a 'safe sex' practice which reduces the risk of catching AIDS.	76.5	18.6	4.9
20 To help stop the spread of AIDS intravenous drug users should be supplied with clean needles.	72.2	19.1	8.7
2 *Statements where there was uncertainty*			
2 I am confident that medical research will discover a cure for AIDS within the next ten years.	29.4	58.7	12.0
21 The AIDS problem is something which is likely to affect me personally in some way in the next fifteen years.	35.3	52.7	12.0
50 People who are infected with the AIDS virus do not have the condition AIDS.	35.7	52.7	11.5
55 During vaginal intercourse without a sheath, there is more risk of infection by the AIDS virus from the man to the woman than there is from the woman to the man.	26.0	51.6	22.3

		% Agree	% Uncertain	% Disagree
35	Voluntary groups within the gay community have made a significant contribution towards fighting the spread of AIDS and helping AIDS victims.	49.4	47.8	2.7
42	It is possible for a woman to have sexual intercourse safely with a man infected with the AIDS provided she avoids contact with his blood and semen.	35.3	46.7	17.9
54	Anal intercourse without a sheath carries a higher risk of transmitting the AIDS virus than vaginal intercourse without a sheath.	44.6	43.5	11.9
53	If a woman orally stimulates the penis of a man with the AIDS virus she runs the risk of becoming infected.	14.7	42.9	42.4
48	It is dangerous to touch or kiss someone who has developed AIDS and is dying as a result.	17.5	33.3	49.2
25	I would be entirely happy to share a cup with someone carrying the AIDS virus.	18.4	32.6	48.9
56	The connection between male homosexuality and AIDS is purely accidental.	9.7	31.5	58.7
3	*Statements where there was disagreement*			
3	The AIDS problem is something which I haven't given much thought to and doesn't really interest me.	7.6	4.9	87.5
31	I'm not concerned that many gay men are dying from AIDS — society is better off without them.	7.6	6.5	85.9
37	I would feel disgusted by explicit descriptions of sexual acts associated with the transmission of AIDS.	6.0	10.9	83.2
24	AIDS is God's punishment for the sin of homosexuality.	4.9	15.2	79.9
41	People who advocate 'safe sex' (practices which carry a low risk of contracting AIDS) are only trying to defend sexual promiscuity.	7.6	16.3	76.0

Table 3.3 Continued

		% Agree	% Uncertain	% Disagree
17	The AIDS epidemic is a warning from God that standards of sexual morality in our society are too low.	8.7	16.8	74.5
36	Reference to certain sexual acts which can pass on the virus (for example, anal intercourse) would not be appropriate in health education lessons in schools.	8.2	18.6	73.2
47	If I were an employer I would feel justified in sacking an employee if I found that he/she had the AIDS virus.	6.0	21.9	72.1
4	*Statements where there was uncertainty and divergence of opinion*			
32	Sexually active lesbian women are less likely to catch AIDS than heterosexual women.	25.7	49.2	25.2
29	So far, the large majority of people infected with the AIDS virus are free from health problems and are not likely to develop full-blown AIDS.	25.0	47.3	27.7
22	Doctors involved in treating AIDS patients run some risk of catching the AIDS virus from them.	25.6	41.8	32.6
38	The only way the AIDS problem will be solved is by a massive movement in society towards stable monogamous relationships.	35.5	32.8	31.7
10	I would be unwilling to give mouth to mouth resuscitation to someone carrying the AIDS virus because of the risk involved in catching the virus.	40.8	31.5	27.7
5	*Statements where there was divergence of opinion*			
5	I would be worried for the health of a child of mine if I knew that a child in his/her class had AIDS.	50.0	16.8	33.2
8	Gay men are to blame for the spread of AIDS.	26.3	27.9	45.9
9	The scale of the AIDS problem is a direct result of the low standard of sexual morality in our society.	44.5	19.8	35.7
13	There are many other health problems facing society which are just as serious as AIDS, for example cervical cancer, heart disease.	44.5	16.3	39.2

		% Agree	% Uncertain	% Disagree
15	I am personally concerned about the possibility of catching AIDS some time in the future.	41.7	23.6	34.6
19	AIDS is the most serious public health problem society has ever had to face.	35.3	25.0	39.7
39	I would be worried about the risk of a child of mine getting AIDS if I knew that one of his/her teachers had the AIDS virus.	31.0	32.8	46.2
46	Haemophiliacs and children with AIDS are more deserving of medical treatment than those who develop AIDS as a result of sexual promiscuity.	37.5	12.0	50.6
51	I find the following statement offensive: 'no fucking without a condom' (*National Student* Magazine, October 1986)	30.4	6.0	63.6
12	I feel I know very little about AIDS.	66.3	9.2	24.4
14	The popular press has used the AIDS problem as an excuse to make sweeping and unjustified attacks on gay men.	52.7	22.8	24.4

In relation to these findings, it should be said that the low levels of endorsement of specifically religious items probably underestimated the extent to which students in the sample made sense of AIDS within a framework of religious belief. A number of them wrote additional comments on the questionnaire suggesting that God has provided people with a clear moral framework for regulating behaviour, and that AIDS is an illustration of what can happen if some choose not to follow Christian teaching. This is illustrated in the following comment by a male student who disagreed that AIDS is either a warning or punishment from God, but who strongly agreed that the AIDS problem 'is a direct result of the low standard of sexual morality in our society:

> I feel that the AIDS problem is not a punishment sent from God, but that it is the natural result of people living in ways which God has told us are unwise manners of behaviour for our own good. He has always had our best interest at heart, and still loves and is concerned about those who are suffering as a result of their own mistaken behaviour, or of someone else's.

A quite different reaction came from a female student who similarly disagreed with the divine intervention items and was uncertain about the issue of moral standards,

> I find it unnecessary and unhelpful to conflate moral and health problems. It is forbidden for Christians to (a) neglect the sick however they may have become so; and (b) attribute any disaster to the judgment of God or see it as a punishment from him for wickedness. 'The greatest of these is Charity' (love).

Sections 2 and 4 of table 3.3 include sixteen items showing the highest levels of uncertainty. Again, these items fall into a number of groupings, the largest of which concerns the question of whether various kinds of social and sexual contact with someone with HIV infection or AIDS carries a risk of infection. Some of the uncertainty reflected here is clearly realistic in the sense that there are issues relating to AIDS which are unresolved. There is no certainty, for example, that a 'cure' for AIDS will be developed, there is no certainty as to how widespread the infection may be by the year 2000, and there is still no certainty about the proportion of infected people who will go on to develop AIDS. Similarly, a high level of uncertainty regarding the risks attached to oral sex is at present reasonable.

Many other issues regarding the nature of AIDS, its epidemiology and modes of transmission are however fairly well established, and uncertainty on these can only reflect lack of exposure to information about AIDS or a lack of understanding. It is clear, for example, that being infected with HIV is not the same thing as having AIDS. It is also clear that risks associated with caring for AIDS patients are so negligible, given proper infection control procedures, as to be insignificant. Similarly, as regards the risks associated with different kinds of sexual activity and contact, it is widely accepted that lesbian sex is probably safer than either male homosexual or heterosexual intercourse, that unprotected anal sex is more likely to result in transmission of the virus than unprotected vaginal intercourse and that the transmission from male to female during unprotected vaginal intercourse is more likely than transmission from female to male.

Finally, one item appears in this list concerned with the contribution which voluntary groups within the gay community have made in educating people and helping people with AIDS. There can be little doubt that this statement is true, and the widespread uncertainty among students in this respect clearly reflects a lack of attention given in the media to the positive and constructive initiatives in self-help mounted within the gay community in response to AIDS.

Sections 4 and 5 in table 3.3 report sixteen items showing the strongest indications of diversity of opinion within the sample. For fourteen of these items at least 25 per cent of the sample agreed and 25 per cent disagreed with the statement concerned. Excluding the five items already discussed in relation to relatively high levels of uncertainty, the majority of items concern two issues: (i) risk assessment and worry/concern over the possibility of infection; and (ii) the 'moral' dimensions of AIDS. With respect to the first issue, there was clear division over the extent to which students would worry about their child coming into contact with someone with HIV infection at school, be they a pupil or a teacher. Differences of opinion were also apparent over degree of personal concern about the possibility of contracting the AIDS virus. Both items included to assess perceptions of the seriousness of AIDS also produced an evenly balanced pattern of response.

With respect to the second area, disagreement was clearly expressed about the role of gay men in the spread of AIDS and the extent to which they have been fairly treated in the media. Students also disagreed over whether the AIDS problem could be attributed to low standards of sexual morality, whether the only solution would be a shift towards monogamy and the idea that some people with AIDS are more deserving of treatment than others (i.e. the so-called 'innocent victims'). All these items in some respect were concerned with whether it is possible to attribute blame for the spread of AIDS in certain directions, either to gay men or to those who are sexually 'promiscuous'.

Two remaining items on 'offensive' language and self-assessed knowledge about AIDS show some division of opinion, but clearly the majority of students did not find the quotation from *National Student* offensive, while a slightly larger majority agreed that AIDS is something they knew little about.

Item Correlations and Elementary Linkage Analysis

Product moment correlation coefficients were calculated for the set of fifty-six items in the questionnaire and, in order to clarify the pattern of association emerging, McQuitty's (1957) elementary linkage analysis procedure was applied. This procedure identified thirteen clusters in

Table 3.4 Ten clusters of items identified by McQuitty's elementary linkage analysis

Cluster name[1] **and items**[2] — **Structure**[3]

A *Homophobia and religious/moral condemnation*
24 AIDS a punishment from God
17 AIDS a warning from God
31 Not concerned gay men are dying
9 AIDS due to low sexual morality
41 'Safe sex' advocates defending promiscuity
8 Gay men are to blame for spread
14 Popular press anti-gay
45 Talk of blame unhelpful
(2 Confident about a cure)

B *Fear, danger and social distancing*
27 Reluctant to sit next to HIV+ person
34 No fear of HIV+ friend
48 Dangerous to touch person with AIDS
1 HIV+ individuals should be quarantined
47 Sacking of HIV+ employee justified
(42 'Safe sex' possible)
(53 Oral sex little risk)
(32 Lesbians less likely to catch AIDS virus)
(43 Some resistance to sheath expected)

C *Worry and non-sexual transmission*
5 Worried about health of child (child)
39 Worried for health of child (teacher)
25 Entirely happy to share a cup
22 Doctors run some risk
10 Unwilling to give resuscitation

D *Sympathy and deservingness*
40 No sympathy for people infected via sex
46 Haemophiliacs more deserving of treatment

E *Education and information/personal concern*
28 'Safe sex' teaching advocated
16 Teaching on avoidance advocated
6 'Explicit' campaign needed
33 Sheath should be advertised
15 Personal concern about AIDS
23 HIV+ having 1+ sexual partners irresponsible
21 AIDS likely to affect me in some way
(11 Sexual behaviour will not change quickly)

F *Monogamy and sexual practice*
28 Social trend towards monogamy needed
44 Sex education should stress monogamy
52 Number of partners not important, practice is
(4 Anyone with 1+ partners runs a risk)

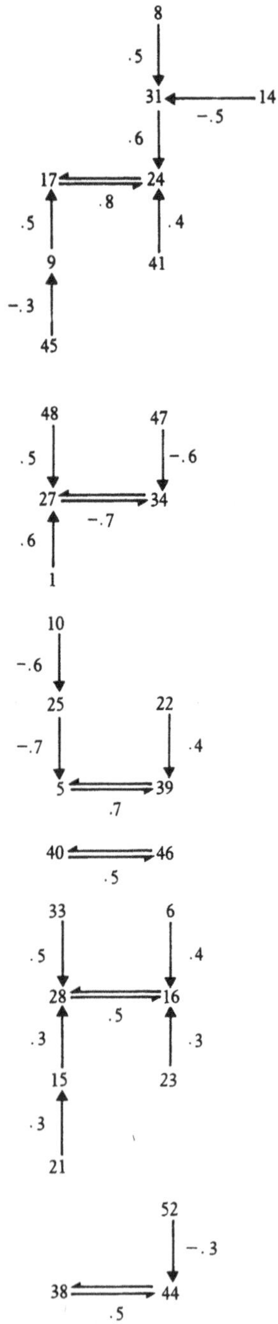

Cluster name[1] and items[2]	**Structure[3]**

G *Seriousness of AIDS*
13 Other health problems as serious
19 AIDS most serious problem
18 Governments bear some blame
(54 Anal intercourse more risky than vaginal)

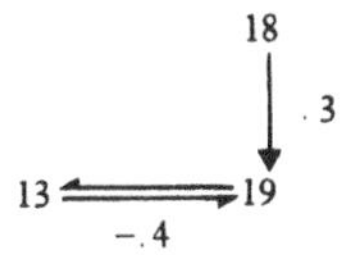

H *Anti-body testing*
7 Blood tests before entry to country
30 Compulsory blood tests should be introduced
49 Insist on blood test before sex

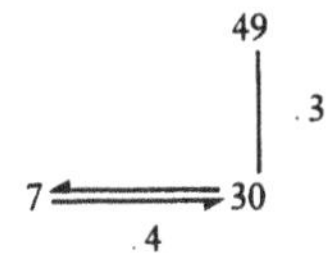

I *Sexual disgust*
37 Disgust over explicit description of sexual acts
36 Reference to anal intercourse inappropriate in schools
51 'no fucking without a condom' offensive
(55 Transmission from man to woman more likely)

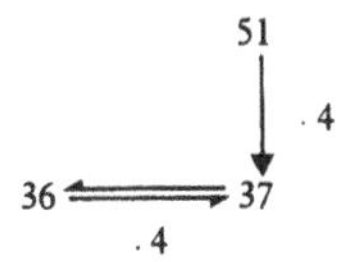

J *AIDS and gay men*
56 Gay — AIDS link accidental
26 Unaffected gay men most at risk

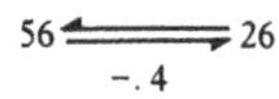

Notes

1 The cluster name is based on the reciprocal pair and those items most closely associated with it.

2 All items associated with each cluster are described in brief. Those with r < ±0.30 are given in parenthesis.
NB: almost all such items concern risk assessments and sexual behaviour.

3 Only items with r ≥ ±0.30 are included in the structural figures. All correlations reported are significant at the 5% level (two tailed).

all and table 3.4 reports the composition and structure of the first ten of these. For each, the reciprocal pair correlation is equal to or greater than ±0.40. The first column reports the items associated with each cluster. Items with correlation coefficients of less than ±0.30 are given in parentheses and, in the interest of clarity, these items have not been included in the structural diagrams. Three clusters (A, D and F) relate to religious and moral attitudes to AIDS, and two clusters (B and C) are concerned with the possibility of transmission in the context of social/non-sexual contact with infected individuals. A further relatively large cluster concerns the need for information and education about HIV infection and AIDS, and is linked with personal concern about being affected by AIDS in the future.

The incidence within the sample of these patterns of response to the questionnaire can be gauged from table 3.3. For cluster A, for example, only a small proportion of students either agree or disagree

Table 3.5 Correlations between reciprocal pair items for clusters concerned with worry/fear and moral issues[1]

Items:	**27**	**34**	**5**	**39**	**17**	**24**	**38**	**44**	**40**	**46**
27 Reluctant to sit next to	—									
34 No fear of contact	−.73	—								
5 Worry for child (*child*)	.60	−.56	—							
39 Worry for child (*teacher*)	.70	−.67	.71	—						
17 Warning from God	.23	−.29	.23	.26	—					
24 Punishment from God	.33	−.36	.30	.38	.78	—				
38 AIDS solved by monogamy	.24	−.31	.18	.29	.41	.38	—			
44 Education should stress monogamy	.07*	−.12*	.04*	.11*	.31	.24	.49	—		
40 Not much sympathy	.24	−.20	.18	.23	.32	.38	.32	.33	—	
46 Haemophiliacs more deserving	.22	−.27	.22	.31	.29	.31	.33	.24	.54	—

[1] All values are significant at the 5 per cent level (two tailed) apart from correlations indicated by *.

with items 17, 24, 31, and 41, and these are surrounded by items characterized by relatively marked divergence of opinion (i.e. items 8, 9 and 14).

In order to examine the interrelationships between the moral and fear/worry cluster in more detail, the intercorrelations between the reciprocal pairs for the five clusters involved were examined. These are reported in table 3.5. It is clear that the items defining clusters B and C are closely related, and in fact, the correlations between the ten main items which define these two clusters show a strong internally consistent pattern. The items defining the moral clusters on the other hand show a looser pattern of association, with links across to the fear/worry items. This is especially true for item 24.

Summated Scales Concerned with Fear/Worry and Moral Issues

On the basis of these results, two summated indices were constructed. The first index concerned with worry, is based on the ten main items included in clusters B and C, and the second, concerned with moral issues, is based on the reciprocal pairs of clusters A, D and F. Figure reports the item-total correlations for the worry and moral indices. It is clear that the total score on the worry scale is strongly correlated with each component item and likewise for the moral index. However, significant correlations are also apparent between the worry index and moral items and between the moral index and worry items. Not surprisingly, the two summated scales are moderately and significantly correlated ($r = 0.45$, $p < 0.05$). Additional items with correlations $> \pm 0.30$ are also reported in table 3.6.

It is interesting to observe that item 1 on quarantining and item 47 on employment discrimination are closely linked to expressed worry and not to the moral index. In addition, two items concerned with compulsory blood tests are also more strongly linked to the worry index. At the outset it has been anticipated that agreement with discriminatory actions and essentially unworkable preventative measures might emerge as a component of 'punitiveness' linked with other 'moral' items. It is clear, however, that endorsement of such items may be more a reflection of worry and lack of understanding or uncertainty about ways in which the virus can be transmitted.

A further trend reflected in table 3.6 is that the items concerned with attitudes towards gay men in relation to AIDS (items 8, 14 and 31) show similar correlations with both the worry and moral indices. In fact, the correlation between item 8 and the worry index is greater than for the moral index. Two interpretations can be offered for this finding. Either those who are not well informed and express more worry about infection via social/non sexual contact are more likely to blame gay men for the spread of AIDS, or those who are homophobic and attribute blame to gay men are more likely to be ill-informed about AIDS and so express more worry. In this respect, it is interesting to observe that a previous study of students' attitudes towards lesbians and gay men conducted at Christ Church College in autumn 1985 (Clift, 1988) suggested that students with more negative attitudes in general towards gay men were more likely to blame them for AIDS. Since homophobia predates AIDS, the second interpretation offered above may be nearer the truth.

Worry, Moral Attitudes and Student Characteristics

Having constructed two scales relating to worry and moral attitudes, it was of interest to examine the distribution of scores on these scales

Table 3.6 Item — total correlations for the 'worry index' and 'moral index'[1]

Items:		**Worry Index**	**Moral Index**
A	*Worry index items*[2]		
1	HIV+ individuals should be quarantined	.68	.32
5	Worried for the health of a child (child)	.81	.28
10	Unwilling to give resuscitation	.69	.40
22	Doctors run some risk	.49	.30
25	Entirely happy to share a cup	.80	.33
27	Reluctant to sit next to HIV+ person	.84	.32
34	No fear of HIV+ friend	.81	.38
39	Worried for the health of a child (teacher)	.83	.38
47	Sacking of HIV+ employee justified	.69	.34
48	Dangerous to touch person with AIDS	.65	.26
B	*Moral index items*[3]		
17	AIDS a warning from God	.31	.72
24	AIDS a punishment from God	.43	.72
38	Social trend towards monogamy needed	.31	.70
40	No sympathy for people infected via sex	.34	.70
44	Sex education should stress monogamy	.13*	.62
46	Haemophiliacs more deserving of treatment	.37	.69
C	*Additional items with correlations of +3 or greater with either index*		
7	Blood tests before entry to country	.39	.15
8	Gay men are to blame for spread	.53	.47
9	AIDS due to low sexual morality	.37	.55
14	Popular press anti-gay	−.40	−.50
30	Compulsory blood tests should be introduced	.31	.11*
31	Not concerned gay men are dying	.49	.50
45	Talk of blame unhelpful	−.35	−.32
23	HIV+ person with 1+ partners irresponsible	.17	.30
41	'Safe sex' advocates defending promiscuity	.25	.36
49	Insist on blood test before sex	.20	.36
56	Gay — AIDS link accidental	−.23	−.31

Notes

1 All correlations reported are significant at the 5 per cent level apart from those indicated by *.

2 All item-total correlations are positive due to rescoring of items. NB. as the index includes all ten items the item-total correlations are slightly inflated.

3 All item-total correlations are positive due to rescoring of items. NB. as the index includes all six items the item-index correlations are slightly inflated.

for the total sample and to explore the connections with student characteristics. The potential range of scores on the worry index is from 10 to 50. Observed scores range from 13 to 49, with a mean of 33.1 and standard deviation of 7.86. The distribution obtained is symmetrical but with larger frequencies towards the upper end of the scale (not worried) than the lower (worried). If scores between 10 and 20 are taken to indicate a consistent level of expressed fear/worry

Table 3.7 Worry and moral index scores and student characteristics

	Worry index				Moral index			
	x̄	**s.d.**	**n**	**t**	**x̄**	**s.d.**	**n**	**t**
Sex								
Men	32.2	8.26	76		21.4	4.61	76	
Women	33.8	7.52	106	−1.36	20.4	4.31	106	1.54
Religious belief								
Religious	32.8	7.93	71		19.0	4.23	72	
Non-religious	33.9	7.50	105	0.99	22.3	3.89	105	5.22*
Political belief								
	x̄	s.d.	n	F	x̄	s.d.	n	F
Definitely right	30.1	6.01	8		18.9	3.64	8	
Right	32.1	6.30	36		19.1	4.38	36	
Centre	31.3	7.85	35		19.7	3.78	35	
Left	34.7	8.19	41		23.3	2.76	41	
Definitely left	39.3	7.57	16	4.19*	24.7	3.97	16	11.98*

* $p \leqslant 0.05$

about contact with infected individuals, then the index identifies eleven students in this position, i.e. about 6 per cent of the total sample. Conversely, scores of 40+ can be taken to indicate a consistent rejection of any need to be concerned about the situations referred to. Thirty students fall in this range of the index (i.e., 16.3 per cent).

For the moral index, scores have a potential range from 6 to 30. Observed scores ranged from 8 to 30 with a mean of 20.8 and standard deviation of 4.45. Again the distribution obtained is fairly symmetrical but with higher frequencies at the upper end of the scale. If scores from 6 to 12 are taken to indicate a consistent and strong moral view of AIDS, then the index identifies seven students in this position, i.e. about 4 per cent of the total sample. Scores of 24+, in contrast, indicate a consistent rejection of a moralizing stance towards AIDS, and seventy-one students fall into this category (i.e., 38.6 per cent).

Data on the relationships between the two indices and five student characteristics are reported in tables 3.7 and 3.8. Sex differences do not emerge for either index, but clear differences between religious and non-religious students are apparent on the moral index. Religious students were more judgmental in general and a small group were singularly punitive and lacking in compassion. A clear trend is also apparent across the five political identification groups with a left-wing political stance being associated with lower levels of worry and moral condemnation. Table 3.8 reports correlations between the two indices

Table 3.8 Correlations between worry and moral index scores and student characteristics

	Worry index		Moral index	
	r	(n)	r	(n)
Sex	0.10	182	0.11	183
Religious belief	0.08	176	0.37*	177
Political affiliation	0.29*	136	0.49*	136
No. sex partners in 12 months	−0.01	155	0.21*	155
Sex preference	0.27*	166	0.26*	166

* $p \leqslant 0.05$

and five student characteristics. It is clear that religious belief, political affiliation, sexual experience and sexual preference are all linked with moral attitudes. Attitudes, with non-religious, left-wing, sexually experienced and non-exclusively heterosexual students being the least condemnatory in their outlook.

Changes Between November 1986 and May 1987

Six months after the initial assessment, the questionnaire was re-administered to seventy-six first-year students in order to identify areas of change in beliefs and attitudes. Detailed results are reported in Clift and Stears (1988), but some of the main findings will be summarized here. Clear and significant changes occurred on nine out of ten of the items included in the worry index ($p < 0.05$), with students being less worried about physical and social contact with infected individuals in the second survey. Some evidence of anxiety about contact with saliva was still apparent, however, and no change had occurred in the extent to which doctors involved in treatment were seen as being potentially at risk of infection.

Students also rated themselves as more informed and were much more likely to know the meaning of the initials AIDS, although only six students could identify what HIV stood for. Less marked though still significant changes occurred on a number of moral/religious items, with there being greater support for the view that a general shift towards monogamy is needed in order to solve the problem of AIDS. For a number of items concerned with the risks associated with specific sexual activities, significant shifts occurred away from uncertainty towards a greater divergence of opinion. For example, in November 1986, 42 per cent of students were uncertain whether oral sex carried a low risk of infection compared with 16 per cent in May 1987. However, levels of agreement and disagreement both increased

Table 3.9 Worry index and moral index scores from first year undergraduates in November 1986 and May 1987

	November 1986			May 1987			
	x̄	s.d.	n	x̄	s.d.	n	t
Worry index	33.9	7.39	85	38.4	5.87	74	−4.33*
Moral index	20.8	4.03	86	20.8	3.98	74	0.03

* $p \leqslant 0.05$

over this period — agreement from 13 per cent to 24 per cent and disagreement from 45 per cent to 60 per cent. Finally, no changes in mean response occurred for three sets of items concerned with sympathy for people who contract the virus via sexual activity, the seriousness of the AIDS problem and the possibility of being directly or indirectly affected by AIDS some time in the future.

It is interesting that despite changes in responses to individual items, especially the worry items, item-total correlations for the worry and moral indices remained consistently high. Table 3.9 reports the results obtained in November and May for the first-year sample on these two scales. The data show a clear shift away from worry over social and physical contact with infected individuals but no change in attitudes towards a range of issues connected with AIDS.

Conclusions

The research reported here is both exploratory and provisional. The sample of students studied is relatively small and in many ways unrepresentative of higher education students in general. It is certainly unrepresentative of the age group concerned. Nevertheless, the present study has achieved three rather different kinds of goals.

As of November 1986, it has served to identify areas of relative consensus, uncertainty and diversity of opinion which are likely to have wider relevance. If relatively well educated young people were uncertain or lacking in understanding on a range of issues, this is surely an indication of widespread uncertainty or lack of knowledge among young people in general.

The research has also identified internally consistent clusters of items concerned with different issues raised by HIV infection and AIDS, and these reflect very clearly the major dimensions underlying reactions to AIDS: lack of understanding, fear, religion, morality and prejudice. Elementary linkage analysis is by its nature elementary, but the results obtained here do offer guidance on ways in which the questionnaire employed can be refined. They also provide pointers to the dimensions which might emerge from the application of more sophisticated multi-variate techniques to data obtained from larger, more representative samples.

Finally, the study has highlighted areas in which positive, unidirectional changes have taken place over the six-month period between November 1986 and May 1987, as well as areas in which changes have been contradictory or non-existent. Not surprisingly, those issues which have a bearing on understanding the nature of AIDS show a clear and consistent pattern of change, but issues involving religious and moral judgment show very little, if any change. Given that issues to do with HIV infection and AIDS are interpreted and understood within a personal framework of religious belief, political persuasion and sexual experience and identity — all relatively stable aspects of individual personality — it is hardly surprising that little change is apparent in these respects.

Beyond the conclusions which can be drawn in research terms from any study, however, there are other issues which should be highlighted in assessing the value of a research project. These include the impact the research has on the people involved (both researchers and researched), the practical implications the results have, and the directions in which the research leads. This project generated a great deal of interest within the college and groups of students and staff were directly involved in the planning and implementation of the research. Those people directly involved clearly gained in terms of their knowledge and appreciation of the issues raised by HIV/AIDS. In addition, the questionnaire itself was generally very well received by students, and many commented that completing it made them realize how little they knew about the subject.

The project has also been significant in relation to our own professional development. This work has resulted in our involvement in local training sessions and conferences for teachers, headteachers and the Kent inspectorate and advisory staff on the issue of education in schools about HIV infection and AIDS. It has also provided the basis for research which is currently underway on the provision of information and education for young people across the South East Thames Regional Health Authority Area (Clift and Stears, 1987). Thus the findings from this study are important not only for the insight they give into undergraduates' beliefs and attitudes, but also for their potential impact on educational policy and practice.

Acknowledgements

The authors gratefully acknowledge the support given to their research by the Principal and governing body of Christ Church College, Canterbury.

Note

1 A copy of the questionnaire used in this research can be obtained from the authors.

References

CLIFT, S. M. (1988) 'Lesbian and gay issues in education: A study of the attitudes of first-year students in a college of higher education', *British Educational Research Journal* 14, 1, pp 31–50.

CLIFT, S. M. and STEARS, D. F. (1987) 'AIDS education strategies for young people', *Education and Health* 5, 5, pp 108–11.

CLIFT, S. M. AND STEARS, D. F. (1988) 'Beliefs and attitudes regarding AIDS among British college students: a preliminary study of change between November 1986 and May 1987, *Health Education Research* 3, 1, pp. 75–88.

JASPERS, F. (1978) 'The nature and measurement of attitudes' in TAJIFEL, H. and FRASER, C. (Eds.) *Introductory Social Psychology*, Harmondsworth, Penguin Books.

MCQUITTY, L. L. (1957) 'Elementary linkage analysis for isolating orthogonal and oblique types and typal relevances', *Educational and Psychological Measurement*, 17, pp 207–29.

PRATT, R. J. (1986) *AIDS: A Strategy for Nursing Care*, London, Edward Arnold.

TAGGART, C. (1986) 'The new puritanism', *National Student*, October, pp. 14, 16 and 18.

4
The Subject of AIDS

Simon Watney

The subject of AIDS is produced and reproduced in a punitive discourse of garrulous morbidity. It has been massively amplified by the powerful institutionalized voices of racism, familialism, nationalism, and a range of deeply-seated anxieties concerning sexual behaviour in general, and homosexual behaviour in particular. In this context, the advent of modern cultural 'theory', with its emphasis on signification, sexuality, 'difference', the unconscious, power, voyeurism, narrative, and so on, seems as fortuitous in its own way as those developments in the fields of virology and immunology which permitted the isolation and identification of the Human Immunodeficiency Virus (HIV) in 1983. Indeed, it could be said that contemporary debates in cultural studies, women's studies, psychoanalytic criticism, textual analysis, the theory of ideology, and so on, have been preparing us for a better understanding of what is now being done — and what is not being done — in the name of AIDS. Yet so far, little by way of deconstructionist analysis has entered the public arena of AIDS commentary. Nor has liberalism yet addressed itself to the question of AIDS with anything like the concern which it has shown for other examples of gross social injustice.

In *The Birth of the Clinic*, Foucault (1975) noted that 'the morbid authorizes a subtle perception of the way in which life finds in death its most differentiated figure'. Within this context it is important to recognize that academics and liberal intellectuals possess no more natural immunity to the effects of 'the morbid' than they have to HIV infection. In this chapter, I will therefore consider some of the ways in which the subject of AIDS sheds light on the political role of modern cultural theory. I will also examine the cultural agenda of

AIDS insofar as it fixes and reinforces a rigid network of heavily medicalized perceptions concerning the gravest matters of potential individual and collective risk. Finally, I will seek to identify the 'other' subject of AIDS, central yet systematically marginalized, the discursively absented Person with the Acquired Immune Deficiency Syndrome (PWA).

It is towards the corrective transformation of the dominant cultural agenda concerning AIDS that the analysis here is directed. For this agenda informs *all* our perceptions of AIDS, no matter how they may be mediated by factors such as class, race, gender and sexuality. No single issue in the modern world is currently more politically loaded than AIDS, and in this arena social policy decisions which will affect and determine all our lives are being proposed, summarily debated, and enacted daily.

The Cultural Agenda of AIDS

The cultural agenda of AIDS relies upon a limited set of heavily overdetermined words and images, any one of which can stand in isolation for the logic of the total structure. It helps contribute a domino theory of the syndrome, which proceeds from the initial notion of 'the AIDS virus' — a phenomenon which it is crucial to recognize as an ideological condensation rather than a medical construction. In making sense of this cultural agenda, we must also distinguish between an infectious disease of the blood (HIV infection), which may be transmitted sexually as well as via direct blood-to-blood contact with an infected person, and the many consequences that this may have. First, HIV may simply lie dormant. Second, it may attack and damage the central nervous system, leading to progressive neurological damage and behavioural change. Third, it may weaken the body's immunological defences, rendering the individual vulnerable to a wide range of AIDS-Related Conditions (ARCs), which are often fatal. Fourth, HIV may so impair the immune system that the body becomes vulnerable to those specific infections and malignancies that result in the diagnosis of AIDS.

The simple distinction between a virus and a syndrome is entirely obscured as soon as the phrase of 'the AIDS virus' is used. At the same time, however, this phrase establishes a basis from which the equally inaccurate notion of 'the AIDS carrier' can be advanced. Thereafter, a discourse comes into being which draws on a rich historical legacy which summons up the all too familiar imagery of contagion and plague. By this time, however, a second condensation has occurred. This collapses together the crucial distinction between infectious and contagious diseases. AIDS is thus presented as if it were indeed a miasmatic condition, with the implication that it can be 'caught' by casual contact.

It is therefore not surprising that 17 per cent of Britons recently polled believe that AIDS can be caught from the seat of a lavatory. But what we should also recognize is that the terms in which such polls are conducted tend only to reinforce prevailing misconceptions. Thus it was recently reported in *Newsday* that 40 per cent of those asked thought that AIDS can be caught by giving blood (Moreno, 1987). What is at stake here is not simply a rational distinction between 'ignorance' and 'knowledge', but the ways in which a specific cultural agenda imposes its values via the very questions it asks. Responses in the *Newsday* poll were triggered by a single question: 'To the best of your knowledge, can a person catch AIDS by giving blood or not?' Readers were then reliably informed that 'the correct answer is no'. The only 'correct' answer to this question would in fact require a challenge to inbuilt implication that AIDS can be caught *at all*. AIDS is a syndrome of at least thirty distinct life-threatening conditions. Of itself, it is neither contagious nor infectious. Thus AIDS commentary effects a remarkable and sinister reversal. Instead of being regarded as threatened, people with AIDS become threatening.

From the notions of 'the AIDS virus' and 'the AIDS carrier' it is a relatively easy syntagmatic slippage to talk of an 'AIDS test'. However, the test referred to here only reveals the presence, or absence, of antibodies produced in response to HIV. Given that these may not be produced for anything up to a year after infection, results from an HIV-antibody test — as it should *always* be described — are highly ambiguous. For even when an individual tests positive and is found to have seroconverted, this does not reveal whether or not she or he will go on to develop neurological damage, ARC or AIDS. Nor does it offer a prognosis concerning which symptoms might appear first. Given that we now know so much about the transmission of HIV, and the ways to prevent it from spreading, it remains to be explained why the cultural agenda of AIDS remains so exhaustively — and exhaustingly — taken up with the issue of testing. By far the most important news in recent months has concerned the seroconversion rate among gay men, which has now fallen to below 1 per cent of those taking the HIV-antibody test in San Francisco and New York (Goldstein, 1987). This signals one of the most astonishing achievements in modern US history. Yet, wherever one looks in the American press — in *The New York Times* or the *Village Voice*, in the *New York Post* or *The Advocate*, the cultural agenda continues to exercise absolute authority. The spectacular success of safer sex campaigning in the gay communities of North America, and the sheer enormity of this achievement as it has been lived through in hundreds of thousands of individual lives, continues to be all but obliterated by an agenda which calls relentlessly for mass testing and/or the quarantine of all those infected.

To understand the force of this forward slippage from the notion of 'the AIDS virus' to the supposed 'remedy' of 'the AIDS test', we need to return to the ways in which the cultural agenda surrounding AIDS has consistently presented the syndrome as if it were an intrinsic property of particular social groups. In this respect, AIDS commentary merely amplifies lay perceptions of health and disease: equating the *source* of an epidemic with its *cause*. According to this view, and following the crudest of retributory logics, the context in which a virus emerges and those first affected are held to be directly responsible for its emergence. Calls for compulsory HIV-antibody testing from general practitioners and other medical professionals thereby demonstrates the profound discontinuity at work between the 'knowledge' generated by epidemiology, and that endemic in other medical institutions.

AIDS is predominantly associated with some supposed 'essence' of those social groups in which it first appeared both in Britain and in the United States. That it should still be so widely regarded as a retributive condition, speaks volumes about the extent to which pre-modern beliefs about disease causation can continue to co-exist with other more scientific understandings. Hence the notion of the 'high-risk group', (which functions as an avatar for 'the AIDS carrier') operates to suggest that certain social groups may of their essence present a risk to others. Admittedly, some commentators have preferred to think in terms of 'high-risk behaviours', and while this term does indeed re-emphasize modes of transmission, it only partially interrupts the relentlessly retributive logic of the overall agenda. Instead of 'risk', of course, we should be talking of 'vulnerability'. Instead of high-risk groups, we should be talking of 'highly vulnerable groups'. Instead of 'AIDS victims', a term which carries connotations of terrorism, we should be talking of people with AIDS. Instead of 'AIDS carriers' we should be talking of people with HIV infection.

Instead of 'the AIDS virus', we should be talking of HIV. And, most importantly, instead of talking about 'compulsory' testing — or as President Reagan put it in 1987 'routine' testing — we should be talking of *punitive* testing.

The dominant cultural agenda clearly invites us to regard AIDS as both a well deserved punishment and a justification for further punitive actions — the latter, rationalized as defence mechanisms against its 'spread'. This is the primary motivation at work within an agenda which endlessly sides *with* the HIV virus in what we are positioned to regard as its purposive mission, to purge the entire planet of the regrettable existence of black Africans, injecting drug users, workers in the sex industry, the 'promiscuous', and, above all gay men. Beyond this identification with the virus, however, lies a still larger unconscious ambition to erase all evidence of the mobility of sexual desire, together with any variation of sexual object-choice beyond the ideal goal of a purely reproductive heterosexuality. If the cultural agenda of AIDS resembles the traditional domino theory of external threat, then this is its internal solution.

AIDS and the Politics of 'Theory'

A colleague recently wrote an article for the British journal *Nursing Times* in which she described the experience of a woman 'living with AIDS'. By the time the piece was printed, an anonymous sub-editor had 'corrected' her words to speak of a woman 'dying from AIDS'. In actions like these, we can observe the cultural agenda of AIDS as it dictates unconscious attitudes, whether at the level of professional 'expertise', or in the form of rumour, gossip, hearsay and jokes. The generating force behind AIDS commentary is, of course, the highly competitive market-place of the multinational mass media industry, for which AIDS is always 'good news' insofar as it promised to increase sales, audience ratings and profit margins. AIDS is thus mobilized to the purposes of an industry which habitually regards its audience as an ideal national family unit, united by child-raising and consumption above all the divisions and complexities of existing social relations. In this manner, the media industry is able to picture itself actively 'serving' and 'satisfying' an audience which it has itself constructed through modes of address which systematically (mis)-represent the entire panorama of the social in the likeness of consumer-spectators who recognize themselves with pleasure in the fantasy space of national family unity. It is in this context that we should recognize the full significance of Foucault's (1979) argument that 'the family' is not the *a priori* object of social policy, but is on the contrary its central and indispensable *instrument.*

Little of the above could have been thought or written when HIV is first thought to have emerged in the United States, at some time in the early 1970s. Since then we have worked our way, with difficulty, through an extraordinary cross-fertilization of ideas to arrive at a mode of theoretical practice which has been alerted by cultural theory to 'what cannot be spoken in what is actually being said' (Rose, 1984). This mode of analysis proceeds from the assumption 'that there is a difficulty in language, that in speaking to others we might be speaking against ourselves, or at least against that part of ourselves which would rather remain unspoken' (*ibid*). Hence we may arrive at the unconscious of AIDS commentary, operating in systematic reversals, in disavowal, and in the most aggressive modes of self-defence. AIDS commentary suggests that throughout contemporary British and American culture, large sections of the population are calmly and routinely regarded in their entirety as disposable constituencies (Watney, 1987). Thus, while a recent British survey suggests that over 90 per cent of the population is in favour of compulsory sex education in schools, another survey reports that a similar percentage of parents is altogether opposed to any kind of teaching about homosexuality. It is from such contradictions that we may learn much about the nature and scale of sexual anxieties and boundaries in both our societies. AIDS evidently threatens the fragile stability of the most fundamental organizing categories for both individual and collective identities, insofar as it raises the reality of sexual diversity.

It seems that both cultures will stop at nothing to prevent the dreadful possibility of sympathetic identification across the chasm of sexual object-choice. Here we may recognize the role of sexuality as the *sine qua non* of modern social organization and control, operating beneath all other levels of gender, class, race and nationality. The political challenge of AIDS lies in the sheer range of issues which it finally obliges us to acknowledge — the sickening ease with which hundreds of thousands of sick and dying people can be cynically dismissed as the supposed agents of their own destruction; the barbarous lengths to which 'modern' and supposedly 'civilized' societies will enthusiastically go to persecute and deny all responsibility for those who are held to threaten 'the family' — an institution and ideological construct from which they are themselves most vigorously and venomously excluded; the sheer volume of hatred and contempt for the marginalized and the oppressed; the question of whether health care is finally a right or a privilege. The degree to which Anglo-American society treats people with AIDS as if they were less than human is the exact and terrifying index of the extent to which both cultures have already been systematically dehumanized. This is not to subscribe to some 'humanist' thought-crime, but merely to observe the bizarre contradiction of a period in which the theoretical diversity of race and sexual object-choice is so endlessly celebrated, while political organizations working on behalf of lesbians and gay men are so lightly dismissed as jejune, or 'essentialist', or merely 'confessional' (Watney, 1986). It should not therefore come as any surprise to discover that the most eloquent analysts of disavowal should themselves ultimately draw attention so clearly to their own psychic defences. The silence of 'theory' on the subject of AIDS speaks volumes for its own resistances.

The 'Other' Subject of AIDS

The 'other' subject of AIDS is the person with AIDS, bound gagged and hidden away behind antiseptic screens and curtains of AIDS commentary, which are occasionally pulled to one side in order to reveal the elaborately stage-managed spectacle of the monstrous. This is the *ne plus ultra* of the cultural agenda of AIDS, the moment at which we are permitted to 'identify' AIDS, and simultaneously denied the possibility of identifying *with* its sufferers. The 'look' of AIDS thus guarantees that it is made visible (and remembered, and dreamed of, and dreaded) as if it were indeed a unitary phenomenon, stamping its 'victims' with the unmistakable and irrefutable signs of the innately degenerate. We thus 'see' AIDS under two guises. First, as 'the AIDS virus', materialized by the technologies of computer graphics and electron microscopy, floating like some alien spacecraft in a dense space of violently saturated colour. Secondly, we 'see' AIDS in living bodies which have been all but stripped of the sensual luxury of flesh, and in faces which are blistered and swollen beyond human recognition. Such images are calculated to appeal to the sadistic. They embody the entire cultural agenda of AIDS at its most concentrated, efficient and revealing. They tell us unambiguously: 'This is what AIDS looks like.' They forbid any further enquiry (Watney, 1988a).

Yet the vast majority of people with AIDS wear no visible stigmata of disease. They go about their lives like everybody else, but with the added burden of a cultural agenda which makes employment, housing, insurance, health care and ordinary social life into a continual and never-ending nightmare. They have been totally leperized. We can only understand the magnitude and significance of this terrible and unrelenting persecution in relation to the position of gay men — who make up by far the majority of people with AIDS — before the epidemic began. Nor are we helped in this situation by the available concepts of 'moral panics' and 'homophobia'. The widespread tendency to regard AIDS commentary as a species of moral panic overlooks the fact that homosexual desire is regarded as scandalous in its totality, and presents moral panic, highly misleadingly, as a discrete and unitary phenomenon (Watney, 1988b). Similarly, the concept of 'homophobia' merely encourages us either to psychologize *all* aspects of homosexual stigmatization, or else to pathologize cultural and historical factors. It is highly unlikely that we shall ever be able to 'explain' the complex domain of attitudes to homosexuality by recourse to a single psychic mechanism. Above all, we must avoid the danger of collapsing together the workings of the social and the psychic. An understanding of the kinds of germ theory that underpin lay perceptions of health and disease can hardly be clarified if we attribute them to the agency of the unconscious, though it should be said that we will not be able to understand how and why they are so widely taken up as sexualized metaphors without the aid of psychoanalysis.

It is precisely in relation to lay perceptions of health that we should begin to develop strategies of resistance to the cultural agenda of AIDS. The simple distinction between infection and contagion, once firmly established, is already a significant block to the internal logic of AIDS commentary. Nor can the facts of the HIV-antibody test be easily digested by those who advocate compulsory (punitive) 'AIDS testing'. In this manner, the 'rhetoric of AIDS' can be forced to speak new meanings. At present it detracts from the security which should come from our knowledge about HIV's modes of transmission and the ways in which infection can be prevented. AIDS rhetoric is therefore a device used by those who would seemingly prefer to see all gay men annihilated rather than contemplate any changes whatsoever in their own sexual behaviour. For although the much discussed topic of a 'possible' epidemic among 'ordinary' heterosexuals is invariably presented on behalf of women and children, it is in fact straight men who are the most threatened — not by HIV infection or AIDS, so much as by the simple use of condoms. At the same time, the rhetoric speaks on behalf of those who would seemingly prefer to see their children die of AIDS rather than let them be 'defiled' by prophylactic education. For there can be no mistake here: AIDS education *is* sex education, and those like Congressman Dannemeyer who oppose safer sex campaigning in America are directly and immediately responsible for the spread of HIV infection and its many consequences. HIV has not yet proved itself to be a respecter of persons. Heterosexual culture can only afford to turn its back on the experience and wisdom of the gay community, achieved from so much pain and suffering, at a truly terrible cost in potential loss of life.

Experience strongly suggests that people cannot be frightened into celibacy, and monogamy is no defence against HIV. It is therefore particularly tragic and regrettable that 1980s America seems to be steadfastly opposed to recognizing that the only way in which it truly leads the world these days is in the example of safer sex campaigns amongst its gay citizens. In Britain, drugs are currently being denied to people with AIDS on the grounds of cost, for the first time in the history of the National Health Service. In America, people with AIDS are being expected to pay to be used as guinea pigs for drug corporations which already make a 300 per cent higher profit on AIDS drugs than on any of their other products (Watney, 1987). It is therefore hardly surprising to find people with AIDS organizing politically in groups such as ACT UP and the 'People with AIDS Coalition' in order to collectively resist the consequences of the cultural agenda of AIDS which I have outlined. If anything can ever teach us about the need to construct new political alliances and identities within and between marginalized groups, it is AIDS. Yet at this moment in time, the entire burden of resisting both the immediate consequences of ongoing social policy concerning AIDS, as well as the cultural agenda of AIDS, falls on the shoulders of those who already have more than enough to deal with in staying well and taking care of their health and refusing to be destroyed by the deafening chorus of hatred all around them, or on those whose lives are spent taking care of them.

Finally it is the image of fatality itself which people with AIDS have done most to challenge. The social identity they have created will be a lasting one, forged in relation to the structures of sexuality, medicine and the state, and demanding both the right to adequate health care and to adequate cultural and political representation. In the long run, people with AIDS' heroic assertion of the intrinsically unremarkable diversity and complexity of human sexuality can only make our cultures stronger and more flexible, insofar as it obliges us all to think more seriously than ever before about the meaning and value of human life. Sooner rather than later we must wake up to the uncomfortable fact that it is only the example of gay men which will ultimately save everyone else's lives. In the meantime we move like Auden's expressive lover, 'To further griefs and greater/And the defeat of grief.'

References

FOUCAULT, M. (1975) *The Birth of the Clinic: An Archaeology of Medical Perception*, New York, Vintage Books.

FOUCAULT, M. (1979) 'On governmentality', *Ideology and Consciousness*, 6, pp 5–23.

GOLDSTEIN, R. (1987) 'State of emergency', *Village Voice*. 30 June.

MORENO, S. (1987) '40% think AIDS can be caught by giving blood', *Newsday*, 16 June.

ROSE, J. (1984) *The Cases of Peter Pan, or The Impossibility of Children's Fiction*, New York, Macmillan.

RUBIN, G. (1984) 'Thinking sex: Notes for a radical theory of the politics of sexuality', in VANCE, C. (Ed.) *Pleasure and Danger: Exploring Female Sexuality*, Boston, MA, Routledge and Kegan Paul.

WATNEY, S. (1986) 'The banality of gender', *Oxford Literary Review*, 8, pp 13–22.

WATNEY, S. (1987) 'AIDS USA', *Square Peg*, 17, pp 28–30.

WATNEY, S. (1988a) 'The spectacle of AIDS', *October*, 43, pp 71–87.

WATNEY, S. (1988b) 'AIDS, moral panic theory and homophobia', in AGGLETON, P. and HOMANS, H. (Eds.) *Social Aspects of AIDS*, Lewes, Falmer Press.

5

Perverts, Inverts and Experts: The Cultural Production of an AIDS Research Paradigm

Meyrick Horton with Peter Aggleton

In this chapter, we will examine the emergence of what can loosely be called an AIDS research paradigm — a set of taken-for-granted assumptions concerning the nature and etiology of AIDS that frames the questions many scientific, medical and social researchers currently ask. In order to do this, we will begin by presenting a typical reading of the phenomenon of AIDS as it is likely to be encountered in the ever growing literature on the subject. This has been generated from an analysis of published serious works on AIDS (as opposed to newspaper articles) and is really a pastiche of that position.[1]

We will then attempt to locate the key ideas generated by this exercise, and hence the image of the person with AIDS, within a larger discourse of disease. In order to do this, we will examine the history of sexually transmitted diseases to identify first, the emergence of venereal disease as a distinct category; and second, the formation of particular images of those afflicted by venereal disease.

Next, we will discuss the construction of male homosexuality, cross-culturally and, within Europe, historically. In doing this, we will identify the role that sexology played in creating homosexuality as a pathological quasi-diseased category. This culturally and historically specific category, along with its later 'inversion' in gay liberation, will be shown to be crucial in the cultural constitution of AIDS as a 'gay plague' in the early 1980s.

Finally, we will try to show how the cultural values identified above operate within the medical model to influence the modern research agenda surrounding AIDS — the kinds of questions that may be asked and the kinds of answers that can be regarded as legitimate. We will conclude by exploring the relationship between the dominant

AIDS research paradigm as it presently is and two other spheres of practice — the larger world of medicine and science, and the popular world that exists outside of AIDS expert journal science.

Our purpose therefore is to sketch out, albeit tentatively, the basis for a more thoroughgoing analysis of a modern thought-style (Fleck, 1979) about AIDS: one enscribed within the collective practice of the scientific community, but one which socially conditions that which may be thought as well as that which may not be debated. In so doing, we will seek to identify some of the psycho-sociological and cultural-historical influences that have contributed to this way of thinking, as well as some of the retentions, embellishments, inversions and transformations of previous modes of analysis it contains.

The 'Just So' Story

There is a kind of a 'Just So' story that is being forged in the vast majority of serious works on AIDS. Perhaps it is unfair to call it a 'Just So' story, since this suggests an almost fictitious stitching up of issues regarding AIDS and its causation along preconceived lines. Nonetheless, it does appear that over the last three years at least, what amounts to a consensus view on AIDS has been constructed which locates its etiology within the dominant biomedical paradigm of germ theory. It should be stressed, however, that the widespread acceptance of this particular mode of explanation may be due as much to the cultural ascendancy of germ theory in medicine (a phenomenon reinforced by the successes of vaccines and anti-microbial drugs post 1940), as to the simple and self-revealing truth of a new virus.

Following Feyerabend's (1975) critique of the history and practice of science, we should be wary of post-hoc rationalizations such as these. HIV was not isolated and identified until long after AIDS had first been diagnosed. The effects of scientific histories of this kind are many and varied, but we should recognize that in this case at least, one result has been to squeeze out from the open arena of debate, alternative accounts of AIDS. Even the implication of a microbe as the cause of AIDS does not *per se* rule out competing or complementary modes of exploration. Nor in fact does it. There are many, often competing, models present in professional as well as lay explanations of the syndrome (Aggleton and Homans, 1987). Furthermore, some of these explanations arise from areas of discourse removed from medical science, though they have informed and, to a large extent, delineated the terrain within which perceptions of health and disease and the manoeuvres of medicine have taken place.

This consensus view can be characterized as follows. In June 1981, the Centers for Disease Control in Atlanta, Georgia reported the cases of five men who had acquired a rare infection called *Pneumocystis carinii pneumonia* or PCP (CDC, 1981). In July, a further report of twenty-six cases of PCP and a rare tumour *Kaposi's sarcoma* (KS), in New York men was published. These two conditions suggested the presence of an underlying immune defect and a new epidemic, the Acquired Immune Deficiency Syndrome (AIDS), was born.

These men happened to be homosexual, and for a while the disease was only seen in gay men. Very soon, however, it was diagnosed in other groups: Haitians, haemophiliacs, injecting drug users and the recipients of blood transfusions. Epidemiologists soon realized that they must be dealing with an infectious agent and used Hepatitis B (a blood-borne viral disease) as a model for infection. A single agent was confirmed when, almost simultaneously, French workers under Luc Montagnier, and American workers under Robert Gallo discovered a virus, called LAV by the French and HTLV-III by the Americans. This novel retrovirus has since been proved to be the cause of AIDS. To avoid confusion, it is now called HIV (Human Immuno-deficiency Virus).

Why Haitians should be at increased risk of developing AIDS seemed at first puzzling until reports from Africa showed that the virus was widespread in some countries south of the Sahara and had probably evolved there from a closely-related green monkey virus. In the mid-1970s, Haitian immigrant labourers brought the virus to Haiti where it was contracted by holidaying homosexuals, who in turn created foci of infection in New York and California. These subsequently contaminated blood supplies.

There are many contestable issues within this scenario which will be returned to later. It is important to recognize though that AIDS, from the outset, was characterized as a member of a larger category of *sexually* transmitted diseases. Hepatitis B on the other hand, a viral disease capable of sexual transmission, is not generally classified as such. Nevertheless, it is effectively transmitted via exactly the same bodily fluids, blood and semen as is HIV, the considered causative virus for AIDS. This essential ambiguity means that AIDS *could* have been categorized differently. Even though its epidemiology was initially modelled on Hepatitis B, it was not characterized as a blood-borne viral disease but as a sexually transmitted disease, the archetype of which is syphilis.

The Venereal Character of AIDS

The taxonomic identification of AIDS as a sexually transmitted disease has profoundly affected popular perceptions of the syndrome and the manner in which people with AIDS are represented. As such, it has firmly located AIDS within the discourse of sexually transmitted disease, one which is indelibly linked to the history of the syphilitic.[2]

The history of the syphilitic is almost 500 years old, and within changing images of the disease one can chart the shifting boundaries of its social construction. The first recorded appearance of syphilis seems to have been during the siege of Naples by Charles VIII of France in 1495 (Cartwright, 1977). The retreating French army spread the disease, as they were a largely mercenary, multinational force, and the 'Morbus Gallicus' soon appeared in the German states. The naming of syphilis thereafter was closely allied to the apportionment of blame. The Neapolitans called it the 'Mal Francese', whilst the French preferred 'Mal de Naples'. The Germans used 'Franzosekrankheit', 'Franzosepocken' or 'Franzosenseuche'. The Flemish and the Dutch considered it the 'Spaanse pokken'. The Portuguese assumed it to be a Castillian disease, while the people of the East Indies and Japan blamed the Portuguese. The Persians accused the Turks. The Poles blamed the Germans, and the Russians unsurprisingly enough accused the Polish. The British, being an island nation, were able to lay the blame on everyone across the water (Rosebury, 1972).

The first representations of the syphilitic appeared on 1 August 1496 in a broadsheet by Theodoricas Ulsenius, illustrated by Dürer. The origin of the disease was assigned astrologically. Most authors assumed that the conjunction of Saturn and Jupiter under Scorpio and the house of Mars on the 25 November 1484 was its cause — benign Jupiter being vanquished by the evil planets Saturn and Mars, and the sign of Scorpio, which rules the genitals, explaining why these organs were the first to be attacked (Bloch, 1901). Astrology also provided a powerful framework of explanation for the new disease, establishing syphilis's venereal character as its first specific difference (Fleck, 1979). From the outset, the syphilitic was characterized as an outsider, an alien tainted by sexual excess — subject to the signs of the Zodiac which determined the 'carnal scourge', yet isolated, deviant and recognizable as such.

In the late fifteenth century, the archetypal embodiment of syphilis was male and portrayed as afflicted, suffering from the pox rather than a herald or bearer of pestilence (Gilman, 1987). Simultaneously however, a retributive portrayal of syphilis also came into being. As Fleck (1979) puts it,

> . . . Religious punishment for sinful lust and sexual intercourse as special ethical significance finally established this cornerstone of syphilology, ascribing to it a pronounced ethical character. . . . Astrology was the dominant science, and religion created the mythical frame of mind. Together these produced that sociopsychological prevailing attitude which for centuries favoured the isolation and consistent fixation upon the emotive character of this newly determined disease entity . . .

It appears likely that numerous other metaphors of disease were subsequently woven into the emergent syphilis complex. By the sixteenth century, there had been a significant remission in the incidence of leprosy in Europe. This left behind empty leprosaria as well as a host of cultural allusions and metaphors which did not remain unused for long. The image of the leper, with its connotations of sickness and pollution, was speedily co-opted into the developing construct of the syphilitic.

During the Enlightenment, the embodiment of the syphilitic shifted from that of the afflicted male, with the unchaste woman being seen as the bearer of the pox. The comparative sexual licence of the eighteenth century saw the young male philanderer as commonplace, indeed almost a required social type, though women were more restrictively described as mothers or wives or whores or mistresses. Interestingly, the etiologic emphasis for the pox was on degree of licentiousness of *practice* as much as it was considered to be located in the licentious woman as source (Bynum, 1986).[3]

As Brandt (1985) has observed, the Victorian period saw the emergence in earnest of the issues surrounding sexually transmitted diseases that are still with us today. Indeed, the essential character of modern institutional forms of medical practice and public health was formed during this period. Two aspects of this are worthy of note: first, the search for 'magic bullets', specific treatments to destroy specific invading micro-organisms; second, major public interventions to control infection. The latter ranged from public health measures requiring doctors to report cases, to calls for obligatory chastity in the military. Within this context, it is worth asking to what extent the professional responses of public health officials and physicians were influenced by medical and scientific advances as opposed to prevailing moral and social concerns. Certainly, since the late nineteenth century, venereal disease has been used to symbolize a society characterized by a corrupt sexuality, as opposed to individual affliction.

Venereal disease came thereby to be socially constructed as an affliction of groups who wilfully transgressed a perceived morality, whether the traditional Christian or the new 'progressive' morality of the nineteenth century secular rationalist. No single agency regulated sexuality, but a variety of bodies of educationalists, physicians and social reformers came to employ venereal disease as a persuasive device for the necessity of a moral probity and a more tightly regulated sexual practice.

But venereal disease traditionally has also symbolically negotiated numerous fears about race, class, gender and particularly sexuality and the family. It has become a vehicle for the rhetoric of prescriptive moral education and reform.[4] The Victorian period saw the elevation of the bourgeois family as a high cultural ideal embodying the virtues of race and nation. Represented in Britain by Queen Victoria and Albert, the family became an enobled (and enobling) institution devoted to child rearing. The home became a private secure place of motherhood, childhood and domesticity. The literature on the evolution of the modern family is large, and many issues within it are hotly contested. Suffice it to say, then as now, the family was an ideological battleground, an arena of dispute since its inception as a middle class cultural ideal.

The perceived threat to the family became an issue of grave social significance for late Victorians, a concern elaborated by physicians when it became accepted that venereal disease posed a unique peril to its existence. It was this period that saw the emergence of 'venereum insontium', disease of the innocent, with congenital syphilis being a tragedy for the exemplary innocent, the child. Women too became innocent sufferers insofar as they could be perceived as morally blameless, as mothers and as upholders of domestic values. The licentious woman on the other hand was of course seen as evil, a perpetrator of affliction as was the profligate man (Brandt, 1986).[5]

The same period saw the transformation of the role of doctors when many became active in the various social hygiene movements formed throughout Europe and America. The concerns of social prophylaxis were those of a heightened morality, and individuals became responsible for protecting themselves and their families from venereal disease. Though social hygiene was remarkable for its unprecedented openness on sexual matters, it nonetheless reinforced the late nineteenth century moral code. In addition, the social hygiene movement was not prepared to leave disease prevention to the possible caprice of particular individuals but rather called on state intervention to encourage, even coerce, people into a correct sense of personal morality (Jones, 1977). Individual morality thereby became a civic duty, and profligate sexuality (in line with degeneracy theory) was perceived as likely to lead to the decline of the race (Rose, 1985).

From the analysis so far, it should be clear that micro-organisms, and the diseases to which they give rise, are socially embodied. This has crucial significance for those who are affected by them. It also has consequences for the ways in which the carriers of disease may metaphorically voice fears about moral and social as well as microbial contagion. Social relations between those who are infected and those who are not, especially when sexual contact is implicated in transmission, thereby become imbued with moral significance beyond that which might be derived from purely scientific considerations. Distinctions between innocent and guilty victims, between those whose actions make it 'reasonable' that they should be infected and those who have acquired infection through 'no fault of their own', operate around many diseases of this kind. These differences are often presented as evidence of a need for moral reconstruction, especially when they are perceived as offering a threat to the family. Thus contemporary demands for a return to the so-called traditional values of chastity before marriage and monogamy within it have a very long history indeed. In many ways it seems as if the advent of AIDS has robbed whole sections of the population of their more rational faculties, encouraging a return to essentially mediaeval (and certainly Victorian) notions of disease, scourge and plague.

But it is not sufficient to understand contemporary responses to AIDS in these terms alone, for they have also been intensely sexualized via processes that link the syndrome to the supposed sexual licence of one key group of actors — gay men. We therefore need to examine how popular understandings of AIDS have been imbued by notions of the 'abnormal' and the perverse which interact with its venereal character.

The Perverse Character of AIDS

Earlier, it was argued that central to modern understandings of AIDS are ideologies that link the syndrome culturally to 'abnormal' and perverse modes of sexual practice. It is within this context that we must analyze some of the ways in which male homosexuality has been used within professional and lay discourse about AIDS. It is for these reasons too that we must try to understand how the contemporary 'AIDS research paradigm' has been imbued with assumptions about the nature and quality of male homosexual desire and practice.[6]

In order to contextualize AIDS within homosexuality, or more properly speaking within the gay community, it is necessary to delineate the historical and social construction of a peculiarly modern phenomenon — men with gay self identities, visible and organized enough to constitute a community with at least one distinctive subculture. In the West, gay men form the vast majority of people with AIDS, and they have been the clear focus of most professional and popular writings on AIDS, from the research journals to the tabloid press.

Whilst it is likely that homosexual behaviour historically has existed and today continues to exist in all societies, it is not culturally universal to define people according to their sexual behaviour. The idea that the homosexual is a distinct social type, necessarily effeminate and inhabiting a characteristic social milieu is of comparatively recent origin (Foucault, 1982). In any attempt, then, (unless one is to be gratuitously essentialist) to survey the cross-cultural, and historical data on the social classification and organization of male homosexual behaviour, an analytical dilemma poses itself: what Murray (1984) calls 'the Scylla of labelling everyone anywhere who engages in homosexual behaviour as a "homosexual" or a "gay person"' versus 'the Charybdis of arguing that there is no category at all'. Whilst there has been, and continues to be, considerable interest in the exotic practices of the other (in academic circles as well as in more popular environments), this fascination does not appear to have revealed an unlimited variation in organizing principles of homosexuality, or heterosexuality for that matter. Relatively few of the conceivable social arrangements for sexuality are actually used by diverse cultures. Murray (1984) (following Adam, 1977) has suggested an ideal type classification of the social organization of male homosexuality based on three forms: age, gender and profession. If one adds gay as a modern variant, this model seems to account for the observed variation in male homosexual social arrangements.

In an age-defined or pederastic social principle, young men are the receptive partners for elder males. This situation is not considered feminizing but is culturally masculinizing for the young male. This situation applies to all men but is transitory. As men age, they take up active sexual roles with both women and younger males. Such systems pertained in Classical Greece (Dover, 1978) and more recently in African Azande culture (Evans-Pritchard, 1970) as well as in Melanesian culture (Herdt, 1984; Gray, 1986).

In gender-defined systems, the receptive partner occupies a perceived female social role and is considered to be feminized by sexual receptivity. This passivo-activo complex is characteristic of the Latin culture of the Mediterranean and of South America, though there are many variations in the form of its social expression (Murray, 1984; Taylor, 1986).

Although modern medical models of male homosexuality define both protagonsits in a homosexual encounter as homosexual, in fact the pejorative labelling of the receptive homosexual as female was retained in the nineteenth century notion of the invert, and is similar to the modern notion of the constitutional homosexual. The other partner is generally thought to be involved in situational homosexuality.

In Europe in the late middle ages, homosexual behaviour was associated with diabolical heresy rather than considered to be the psychological or physical property of particular individuals. Sodomy referred to all unnatural acts as defined by the edicts of the church. A transformation to gender-defined notions of male homosexual behaviour only took place sometime in the late seventeenth century. Bray (1982) charts the appearance of the effeminate subculture of the 'molly culls' at the beginning of the eighteenth century. His work shows that in England anyway, gender defined homosexuals existed before the advent of the 'medical model'. It is with the rise of this model though that the modern male homosexual appears in earnest.

The nineteenth century was the great age of armchair taxonomy where Darwin provided the metaphor which allowed the exploration and definition of every conceivable species and sub-species of human existence. The quasi-medical discourse of sexology was born which typologized and colonized the exotic sexual areas of human behaviour as perversions and deviations. Weeks (1977, 1981 and 1985) has admirably traced the formation of this discourse, its embodiment within the 'medical model' and the way in which sexology was able to establish a terrain within which all subsequent debates around sexuality were obliged to manoeuvre. This review of sexology is critical in that it shows the ways in which homosexuality was posed as a disease state with an imagined (although always undiscovered) specific etiology. This is crucial in understanding the placement of

AIDS within the prior disease model of homosexuality and the way in which the former has cognitively patterned the latter. Particularly noteworthy is the way in which sexology has placed the 'origins' of homosexuality alongside its cause as if they are coterminous. This clearly resonates with the contemporary situation where the perceived origins of AIDS in Africa is often considered equal to its cause.[7]

If medicine has never been sure of the cause of male homosexuality it has certainly been convinced of its pathology. In Britain and the United States, homosexuality was not removed as a mental illness until the mid-1970s, and then only under considerable pressure from gay activist organizations (Weeks, 1985).

Foucault (1982) however, in his rejection of 'the repressive hypothesis' has argued that the eighteenth and nineteenth centuries were not a time of simple repression, prohibition and coercive control. Rather, they witnessed an expansion of a discourse of knowledge/power and an extension of rationality to hitherto unexplored social and psychological domains via the overpowering desire to name and control. *Scientia sexualis* constantly multiplied the discourse around sexuality, but whilst generating greater control, it equally generated greater resistance to its power.

> . . . There is no question that the appearance in nineteenth century psychiatry, jurisprudence, and literature of a whole series of discourses on the species and sub-species of homosexuality, inversion pederasty, and 'psychic hermaphroditism' made possible a strong advance of social controls into this area of 'perversity'; but it also established the preconditions for a 'reverse' discourse: homosexuality began to speak on its own behalf, to demand that its legitimacy or 'naturality' be acknowledged, often in the same vocabulary and using the same categories by which it was medically disqualified . . . (*ibid*)

Yet while the works of sexual reform pioneers such as Ulrichs and Carpenter may indeed have been produced by this 'reverse' discourse, their effects were limited, and the advent of law reform in the 1960s was not simply a relaxation of legal restrictions regarding male homosexuality but rather a matter of changing definitions of the law. In Britain for instance, law reform following the *Wolfenden Report* resulted in the distinction between consenting adults in private, and the public sphere. This did not mean that male homosexuality was accepted by society, rather the focus of its control was shifted. In fact this meant that policing of the public arena could be extended (Weeks, 1977 and 1981).

The gay liberation of the 1960s and 1970s did not occur as the result of the floodgates being opened by liberal law reform. Gay activism and gay identity were the result of longstanding social processes involving both definition and self-definition. However, the event that symbolically generated a coherent consciousness of a gay movement occurred in June 1969 when the police, in routinely raiding a gay bar, the Stonewall Inn in New York, met determined resistance (Altman, 1974; Weeks, 1977). In a sense it is still too soon to tell what the full consequences of Stonewall have been, but in the intervening years, gay and lesbian groups organizing as such have had many successes in building a community — newspapers, publishing houses, welfare organizations, non-commercial meeting places, police monitoring groups, as well as numerous commercial venues.

Unfortunately what mainstream society sees is something quite different. It has perceived the growth and diversification of a pleasure class, imagining gay men given over to the pursuit of their own sex. Of course, gay men themselves are a product of particular cultural forces, and to some extent partake of the same vocabulary. If gay men have been constructed as a unique species, as distinct and inherently promiscuous, it is not surprising that some should internalize and act upon this view. Moreover, consumerist values have packaged a gay lifestyle, and gay men attempting to escape oppression have been assimilated into economic and cultural upward social mobility. What notions of a decadent lifestyle do not see is that consumerism of this kind depends on a *repression* of sexuality, with continuing demand being dependent on people remaining dissatisfied with what they have. But whilst a burgeoning gay subculture has emerged in parts of Europe and the United States, it must not be assumed that this has met with easy tolerance. In the United States there are anti-homosexual statutes in more than half of the member states of the Union, and in both Europe and the United States there are frequent calls for the recriminalization or extended regulation of male homosexuality.[8]

Moreover, it is vital to recognize that here, as in other matters, care must be taken to distinguish fiction from reality. An understanding of the prevalence of male homosexuality (even based on Kinsey figures) has to show that most gay men do not live in London, New York or San Francisco. In fact the vast majority of gay men are isolated in rural areas or urban environments where there is likely to be little by way of an organized 'gay scene'. In this kind of situation, opportunities for same sex relationships are likely to be severely limited. But it is not what people do that is fundamental in constructing a culturally formed thought-style, but what they are perceived as doing.

Re-reading the Story of AIDS

If it is accepted that contemporary discourse around male homosexuality (itself bounded by the practices of medical culture), has a particular place in the cognitive terrain of a modern scientific thought-style, it should come as no surprise to discover that the first reports from the CDC in 1981 of cases of PCP and KS recognized the 'essential' and significant homosexuality of the men with these conditions. This is not to imply a form of cognitive determinism — after all, over 90 per cent of the early cases diagnosed were amongst a sub-set of gay men attending clinics for the treatment of sexually transmitted diseases in large urban areas, and their sexuality would have been reported to the CDC as a matter of course.

That the sexuality of people presented with a novel disease should be immediately apparent, it is argued, stems from the organization of gay men in urban concentrations following the emancipation movement of the 1970s and the growth of public awareness of such a community. Medical reports dealing with venereal disease prior to gay liberation often talked of examination revealing unsuspected homosexual tendencies. A New York physician in a busy gay practice in the 1980s would hardly be so 'unsuspecting'.

That an immediate association between 'the gay lifestyle' and a fatal syndrome indicating an underlying immune deficiency should be made has everything to do with the social and cultural formation of the notion of the 'promiscuous homosexual' and his 'innate pathology'. One of the first reports from the CDC (CDC, 1981) remarked that 'Two out of the five (cases) reported had frequent homosexual contacts with various partners', and further that 'the fact that these patients were all homosexuals suggests an association between some aspect of a homosexual lifestyle or diseases acquired through sexual contact and Pneumocystis carinii pneumonia in this population'. These connections were further consolidated by the use of the category Gay Related Immune Deficiency (GRID) as an initial description of the condition. Those affected were thereby located simultaneously within the stigmatized frame of reference of a culturally specific category relating to sexuality and within the bounded frame of reference of terminal disease. This emerging homosexual/disease complex is prefigured by the pre-AIDS 1970s medical concepts by Gay Bowel Syndrome and Gay Bar Syndrome (Johnson and Ho, 1985).

The CDC thereafter has consistently constructed the epidemiology of AIDS according to 'risk group' criteria. By 1983, these groups included homosexual and bisexual men, injecting drug users (usually inaccurately referred to as intravenous drug users), haemophiliacs, Haitians and the recipients of blood transfusions. These 'risk groups' were intended to reflect populations linked by the incidence of AIDS though of course the term suggests far more by implying that these same groups might be a risk to the population as a whole. The argument here is less that the term 'risk group' is open to abuse but rather that it fundamentally misrepresents the nature of AIDS and the modes of transmission of HIV, resulting in the assumption that all gay and bisexual men are at equal risk of developing AIDS and, by implication, the view that heterosexuals are at no (or greatly reduced) risk.

It is noteworthy that under political pressure Haitians were removed as a 'risk group' from surveillance reports (as early as August 1983 in New York). In 1985, the CDC remarked that 'the Haitians were the only risk group that were identified because of who they were rather than what they did' (cited in Altman, 1986). The same could be said for gay men. What is at issue here is whether there are intrinsic risks for developing AIDS by belonging to a given population. Given what is now known about the way in which HIV is and is not transmitted, it is clear that it is certain *practices* which place an individual at risk, not the simple membership of a community. It would therefore make more sense to categorize individuals according to their homosexual or bisexual behaviour, as in fact does the Canadian Laboratory Centre for Disease Control, than on the basis of their socio-sexual identification.

This does not mean that the epidemiology as it presently exists is wrong, but there are other ways of representing the situation. In 1987, 30 per cent of people with AIDS in the United States were black or hispanic (50 per cent of whom are heterosexual). In the same year, a black woman was thirteen times more likely than a white woman to develop AIDS in the United States, and 92 per cent of perinatally acquired cases of HIV infection were in black or hispanic children (Goldstein, 1987). In effect, in America there is one disease divided by two cultural moments: first, the AIDS of largely middle class fairly well organized gay men and second, the AIDS of the fragmented, the poor and the oppressed — what clearer indication can there be of the political economy of health?

Epidemiology is sociologically interesting precisely because the classifications it uses not only reflect prevailing thought-styles but help establish modes of thinking and doing around AIDS which condition strategies of response. In September 1985, for example, the United States government calling on its experts in an attempt to control the rising 'epidemic of fear' which had resulted in, among other things, mounting school boycotts, felt able to reassure its citizens that panic was inappropriate because AIDS remained confined to the gay and injecting drug using populations (Krieger, 1987).

But this thought style has implications beyond epidemiology. In particular, it has consequences for the way in which issues to do with AIDS are reported in medical and scientific journals and the way in which these same issues are subsequently taken up and used. In the remainder of this chapter, we will attempt a re-reading of a number of articles taken from the early scientific and medical journal literature on AIDS to show how the concerns identified above inform the analyses offered.[9] In particular, we hope to identify how the events they describe are framed by an agenda which ascribes primacy to the venereal and perverse character of AIDS — moreover, one which establishes well defined roles for those at threat and those who threaten. The cast consists unsurprisingly enough of the rigidly characterized heterosexual (probably white) majority on the one hand, and on the other, the promiscuous (and probably drug using) homosexual supported by the black, generally promiscuous (and often homosexual) African.

The first article we will look at is by B. Frank Polk from the Johns Hopkins School of Hygiene and Public Health in Baltimore. It was originally published in the *Journal of the American Medical Association* with the title 'Female to male transmission of AIDS' on 13 December 1985. In response to previous articles debating female to male transmission, the author writes:

> . . . Fortunately for human society, these authors are probably incorrect in suggesting frequent female to male transmission of HTLV-III/LAV. No data are currently available to support the contention that this virus is spread sexually from women to men . . . The African observations are subject to misinterpretation. In

> Africa the male to female ratio of observed AIDS cases is very nearly 1 : 1 . . . Heterosexual promiscuity is very common in sub-Saharan Africa, while homosexuality is said to occur rarely, although no valid data about homosexual activity are currently available. These simple observations have led many to infer that bidirectional heterosexual transmission is a major mode of virus transmission in Africa. This association may be greatly confounded by the medical re-use of inadequately sterilized needles and syringes for administering therapy for the sexually transmitted diseases that are causally associated with heterosexual promiscuity . . . The level of alarm over this pandemic is substantial and appropriate. We should not raise that level with conjecture about female to male transmission, but should embrace the null hypothesis . . .

Clearly the concern here is to prevent an escalation of alarm (even though the author feels that the current level is 'appropriate') by reassuring people that heterosexual sex poses no risk unless it is tainted by promiscuity. Then, and in connection with treatment for sexually transmitted diseases, contaminated needles may transmit the infection. Though of course there is properly speaking a risk associated with HIV contaminated needles and syringes, this could hardly be the major risk factor, in Africa or anywhere else. The cultural allusions here are clear — promiscuity, venereal disease, the suggestion of undisclosed homosexuality (for if female to male transmission is denied, then infected men must acquire HIV from other men) and the improper use of syringes — improper, both because of a lack of medical hygiene and because of the suggestion of impropriety due to their use in the treatment of promiscuously acquired infections.

The next article is by Nancy Padian from the School of Public Health at the University of California, Berkeley and John Pickering from the University of Georgia. Entitled 'Female to male transmission of AIDS: A re-examination of the African sex ratio of cases', it appeared in the *Journal of the American Medical Association* on 1 August 1986. The authors state:

> . . . Sexual transmission (of HIV) from females to males is less well documented. Although we do not doubt that this phenomenon occurs we question whether the ratio of male to female cases in Africa necessarily supports the hypothesis that AIDS is primarily spread in Africa by bidirectional heterosexual transmission . . . the high ratio of male to female AIDS cases

> in the United States can be explained largely by sexual transmission amongst homosexual and bisexual men . . . In contrast few cases in Africa are attributed to homosexual contact, a finding that could be based on fact, but that could also reflect cultural or methodological biases in interviewing techniques . . . The 1 : 1 sex ratio in AIDS cases can be explained without invoking female to male transmission. The low African ratios could be explained by a higher proportion of bisexual compared with homosexual men in Africa than in the United States . . . If few males are exclusively homosexual in Africa and if most homosexual behaviour is amongst young bisexual males, then bisexual males could be largely responsible for the transmission of AIDS. In this case, if every bisexual male had an equal number of male and female partners . . . then the observed sex ratio of cases could be close to unity with little or no female to male transmission . . .

This paper attempts to explain African AIDS sex ratios entirely by recourse to homosexual behaviour. Whilst it would be foolish to claim that homosexuality does not exist in Africa, even a casual consideration of Africa as a continent in its own right (rather than as a backdrop for Californian ruminations) would reveal the massive cultural differences in the organization and perception of male same sex behaviour throughout sub-Saharan Africa. To suggest that the vast majority of African men are so mathematically bisexual that they have strictly 'equal numbers of male and female partners' is a cultural nonsense.

In fact, papers like these are rarely interested in Africa. There is no attempt to systematically explore the epidemiology from an understanding of African cultural diversity, which would show if anything it is the urban middle class who are most at risk. Instead, we have the Anglo-American category of homosexuality used as a cognitive halter to restrain the thought-style of scientists and physicians. Whilst the rigidly policed categories of mutually exclusive sexuality might appear to be more flexible in this paper in that it is inferred that homosexual behaviour might be practised by equally heterosexual men, the boundaries have been extended just for Africa, leaving American heterosexuality as marked off (and safe) as ever.

Such an analysis is sustained by another paper in the 1 August edition of the *Journal of the American Medical Association*. 'Heterosexual transmission of AIDS' by Richard B. Pearce of San Francisco is a reply to a previous article discussing the possibility of heterosexual transmission. Its author states:

> . . . Because there are no data to indicate that 'soldiers are more likely to lie (about homosexuality or IV drug use) than civilians', Redfield *et al.* conclude that they are telling the truth. Unfortunately the mere absence of data to the contrary does not by itself make the opposite assertion true . . . We are given the conclusion that HTLV-III is a 'bidirectional sexually transmitted disease' which the authors find in 'non-drug using, strictly heterosexual men' . . . While it is true that in Africa, the incidence of AIDS . . . is nearly equal among men and women, we ought not to automatically assume that heterosexual transmission of the AIDS virus is likely here. Parasitic disease has been found repeatedly to be a risk factor for seropositivity to the AIDS virus or AIDS itself in Africa and Venezuela, and for seropositivity to HTLV-I in southern Japan, Africa and Venezuela . . . Parasites are prevalent in Haiti and amongst Haitian immigrants to the United States. Surveys worldwide place the prevalence of intestinal protozoa in homosexuals at approximately 60 per cent. Parasites are both immunosuppressive and mitogenic for T-cells and may easily explain the restriction of opportunistic retroviruses to primates and humans with parasites and those living in the tropical regions. It is not improbable that a virus might infect 'bidirectionally' in Africa but does so only rarely in the United States . . .

This article appears more than a little confused as the author obviously subscribes to a multifactorial view of AIDS. However, in an attempt to have it all ways, HIV (then known as HTLV-III) becomes both an immunosuppressive agent (as a co-factor) and an opportunistic infection in the immunocompromised. But more informatively, we have the linking of parasites, monkeys, Africans, Haitians and homosexuals — the parasitized and the perverted! Whilst the paper posits a different explanation for AIDS in Africa, it operates with the same apparent need to explain away the possibility of heterosexual transmission: the implication being that in the West, men claiming to have contracted HIV infection heterosexually (especially if they are in the armed forces) are probably lying.

Finally we will examine a paper from the journal *Neurology* by F. Flynn, E. Popek and M. Maccario from San Francisco.[10] It is a case study describing a 'Change from homosexual to heterosexual behaviour during a seizure in a patient with the Acquired Immune Deficiency Syndrome'. The authors state:

> . . . Changes in sexual drive and preference have been described in brain injury, seizures and after temporal lobectomy. Heterosexual behaviour developing during a seizure in a previously neurologically intact homosexual has not previously been reported . . . A 58-year-old man with AIDS who had no previous history of heterosexual behaviour approached a female while in mixed company and attempted sexual intercourse with her. This was followed in minutes by a right focal motor seizure with secondary generalization. Over the next few hours, three additional stereotypic seizures occurred. CT was normal. EEG demonstrated a left frontotemporal focus. On phenytoin, the patient had no further seizures. The patient resumed strict homosexual behaviour. A few months later, the patient died from necrotizing bacterial pneumonia. The brain at autopsy demonstrated diffuse subacute encephalitis caused by cytomegalovirus (CMV) . . . The neural substrate of homosexual behaviour remains unknown. However, there appears to be a similar propensity for sexual preference change in homosexuals as in heterosexuals when there is dysfunction of the frontotemporal or limbic areas . . .

This makes chilling reading indeed. Rich in metaphor, the article is at first sight only peripherally interested in AIDS. In fact, as a more careful examination reveals, AIDS here speaks so directly of homosexuality that it appears, as is often the case with long used metaphors, as a metonym for it. It is extraordinary though that the focus of concern in this paper lies not with the patient's very real suffering in the final stage of a terminal illness, but with the possible neurophysiological basis of his sexuality. This palpably reflects continuing medical interest in the cause of homosexuality and speaks volumes of an essentialist view of sexuality. As for the claim that the patient had a sexual preference change because he approached 'a female while in mixed company', this offers a particularly unappealing view of heterosexuality, which it defines strictly according to opposite sex object-choice and a fit induced assault! It is almost as if sexuality is little more than a variety of encephalitis. According to this mode of analysis, the boundaries of the distinct sexual types are so deeply enscribed in the nervous tissue of people that it requires a major seizure to re-align them.

Some General Characteristics of the Emergent 'AIDS Research Paradigm'

Throughout this chapter we have tried to identify some of the taken-for-granted assumptions concerning the nature and etiology of AIDS that frame the research agendas of scientific, medical and social researchers. These help constitute a unique thought-style — an interwoven network of 'facts' about AIDS that gains solidity via its socially reproduced tenacity. But thought-styles are cultural phenomena, and are reproduced and transformed by the interplay between different groups of actors. In Fleck's (1979) preliminary analysis of the structure of scientific thought-styles, he found it necessary to distinguish between thought-styles themselves and those who communally carry them — the thought-collective. He further separated out the thought-collective of science into an esoteric circle of experts surrounded by a large exoteric world. Within the esoteric circle there is a core of elite experts. Similarly, the exoteric world is divided, with a more practically oriented sector lying close to the esoteric circle. Entry to the world of experts is gained by initiation through a scientific education. In consequence, there are four forms of science, each with its own particular literature — journal science for the elite core, *vademecum* or handbook science for the standard experts, popular science for the exoteric circle and textbook science that allows for initiation into the esoteric world.

Ideas like these can be adapted to form the basis of an analysis of the thought-styles that characterize the modern AIDS Research Paradigm. A preliminary model of the thought-collective of the AIDS world is shown in figure 5.1. The structure of the model is hierarchical, imaged as a pyramid or a cone, with lines of dominance from the apex down. The lower levels, though cognitively inferior, provide necessary support for the higher levels in the manner of a pyramid. The esoteric thought sphere is therefore both influenced by and dependent on the lower levels. The base of the pyramid provides the ultimate cognitive restriction and consists of 'that which is not debated'. Constraint by this level is applied passively in that within a given thought-style certain things are rendered unthinkable. Much of this chapter has been concerned with identifying some of the key constituents of this base. Thought changes, either within a structure over time, or by individuals moving between thought-styles; though it should be noted that generally speaking communication only takes

Figure 5.1:

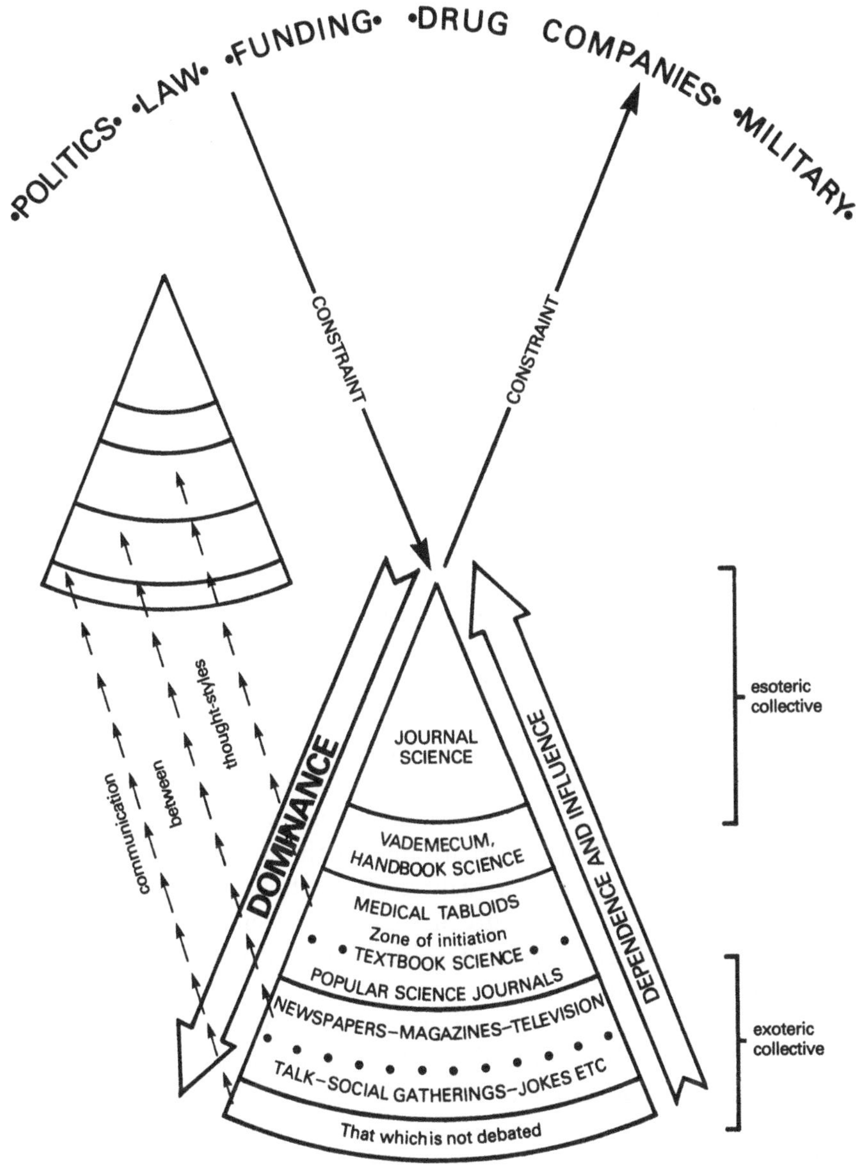
•POLITICS• •LAW• •FUNDING• •DRUG COMPANIES• •MILITARY•
CONSTRAINT
CONSTRAINT
communication
between
thought-styles
DOMINANCE
DEPENDENCE AND INFLUENCE
JOURNAL SCIENCE
VADEMECUM, HANDBOOK SCIENCE
MEDICAL TABLOIDS
Zone of initiation
TEXTBOOK SCIENCE
POPULAR SCIENCE JOURNALS
NEWSPAPERS–MAGAZINES–TELEVISION
TALK–SOCIAL GATHERINGS–JOKES ETC
That which is not debated
esoteric collective
exoteric collective

place between the lower levels. The elite core is both practically and cognitively incommensurate with other elite journal worlds, and the pyramid as a whole is located within a further dome of constraint constituted by the world of politics, of finance and funding.

One of the advantages of this particular model is that it does not seek to reduce the thought-collective around AIDS to the organizational structure of a community. It therefore allows for an analysis of tensions within and between groups of individuals as members of a thought-style. It also highlights the importance of enquiry into the processes that take place at different levels. It would be interesting, for example, to explore the processes of decontextualization and recontextualization that take place as research findings (and the ideologies that operate within them) move from the world of journal science to other spheres. In particular, the role of popular medical journals — the medical tabloids — is worthy of particular study. Journals such as *Hospital Doctor*, *Pulse*, *General Practitioner* and *Doctor* are in one sense part of the esoteric self-referring world of the medical expert, yet in many respects their style is surprising. Issues are often sensationalized within them in a direct parallel of media reporting in the national tabloid newspapers. Headlines such as 'Russians come out of closet in joint AIDS talk'[11], 'AIDS ignorance is bliss for gays'[12] and 'Prostitutes run for cover as fear of AIDS strikes'[13] are not untypical. These journals, and the manner in which they consolidate the commonsense that doctors operate with, are clearly worthy of more detailed study.

In the space available here we can do no more than begin to identify a programme for future enquiry. Central within this will be research into the manner in which the category 'AIDS' is taken up and used. Already we can see in arguments about the extent to which heterosexual transmission is a reality, efforts both to heterosexualize the phenomenon and to capture it for a moral and political agenda that seeks to privilege so-called traditional sexual values and patterns of behaviour above others.

As stated above, thought within a given thought-style is formed and changes both diachronically and synchronically. Earlier in this chapter, we were concerned to sketch out the evolution of the concept 'AIDS' by recourse to the historical development of understandings of disease and sexuality that have structured the way in which the syndrome is thought of and spoken about. Perhaps the most unhelpful notion in analysing this kind of cultural evolution is that of 'natural selection'. In its Social Darwinistic incarnation, this assumes that emergent or newly-involved concepts, theories or even paradigms, replace prior existent forms with better, and 'fitter', explanations. The concept of thought-styles, however, enable the development of an epistemology that allows the recognition of the vestiges of previous modes of understanding as well as an analysis of how they influence a contemporary ascendant style. This has been shown to be crucial to understanding the formation of 'AIDS' as a historically shaped thought-style. What may be less clear is the way which this thought-style is sociologically and cognitively structured contemporaneously. The purpose of the model then is two-fold. First, it seeks to offer an explanatory model of the kinds of ways in which thought-styles are constructed and in turn themselves construct thought. Second, it seeks to indicate further avenues of enquiry that could corroborate this. It is proposed that the mode of investigation of a thought-style should be both epistemological, in terms of analyzing the structures and products of a thought-style, and sociological in terms of examining the formation of a fairly stable thought collective or community. At the present time, a number of key arenas of investigation can be identified. These include the arenas of discourse production and reproduction, the arena of the texts and the arena of discourse regulation.

The Arenas of Discourse Production and Reproduction

These arenas may be studied sociologically. For instance, the circles of influence around intellectual leaders within a thought-collective are not coterminous with the formal hierarchies of a community's institutional form. In this light, international conferences become important ethnographically the patterns of association between those who attend them are crucial for the production and reproduction of AIDS knowledge. Within this context, dinner parties, academic soirees and networks of friendship among members of a thought-collective may be equally important points of articulation for the esoteric circle as are conference papers themselves.[14]

Medical education too plays a key role in reproducing dominant understandings of AIDS, and the way in which 'AIDS' is now taught in this context is clearly critical. Given the *rites de passage* associated with initiation into a thought-style, it can lay structures of thinking within a thought-style that become indissoluble subsequently. Ethnographic research would surely pay dividends here.

The Arena of the Texts

Here, a comparative epistemological study needs to be elaborated in which the socio-intellectual characteristics of the differing textual worlds comprising the AIDS research paradigm are examined. Here, a few tentative suggestions only can be made. These will focus on the important distinctions to be drawn between journal science, *vademecum* science, popular science and textbook science.

Journal science, the world of the esoteric experts, is a form of personal exchange whereby elite members signal the possible entry of new 'facts' into the established world of science. By way of contrast, *vademecum* or handbook science is clearly a more authoritative discourse. Inclusion in this world, which is intended for general experts, signals the consolidation of knowledge. Already, the form of its production and its controversies have been lost. Popular science is a highly complex social field. These texts, intended for the 'educated amateur', offer a clear authoritative voice from the thought-collective. The critical division this sphere marks out is that beween expert and popular knowledge. The epistemology of this kind of popular knowledge is understudied but clearly needs to be elucidated. Textbook science, on the other hand, represents the zone of initiation into a thought-style. In 'AIDS' knowledge, this area needs to be closely observed. Readers on AIDS as introductory texts are increasingly appearing. The general form that these textbooks take is authoritarian. They serve to induce the novice into a *Weltanschauung* in which not only are old or commonsense facts viewed differently, but new ones actually appear. The content of these texts reveals the 'evident facts' of a given thought style. An analysis of textbook science is therefore likely to indicate the dominant features of the emergent AIDS research paradigm.

The Arena of Discourse Regulation

This particular area is worthy of investigation both sociologically and empirically since the sites of operation of AIDS knowledge have an intricate role in mediating and consolidating the thought-style. In this sphere, for instance, the numerous agencies dealing with HIV and AIDS education, counselling and treatment are located. Bodies with an educational role are likely to repay study because it is within them that the 'facts about AIDS' are reconstructed and processed for dissemination. In the United Kingdom, sexually transmitted disease clinics are a crucial area of the thought-collective of AIDS practice.

Ethnographic enquiry into their operation would be particularly illuminating, since practice is epistemologically imbued (see Silverman's chapter elsewhere in this book). Similarly, the counselling agencies, both orthodox and heterodox, should be explored. How the person with HIV antibodies, AIDS Related Complex or AIDS is counselled, for example, reflects the contribution not only of the AIDS thought-style but also the thought-styles of counselling and bereavement. Hospice care of people with AIDS should be viewed, for instance, for the significance of its own thought-style which, among other things, signals modern notions of good and bad death. This reframes medical notions of the fatality of AIDS within a larger discourse of death and dying.

Throughout much of this enquiry, a dual approach of comparative epistemology and sociologic enquiry will need to be adopted, because as Fleck (1979) has noted,

> . . . The general structure of a thought-collective entails that the communication of thoughts within a collective, irrespective of content or logical justification, should lead for sociological reasons to the corroboration of the thought-structure.

In this chapter, we have tried to identify some of the key components of a more integrated approach to the understanding of AIDS — one that sees the formation of the concept 'AIDS' as a bio-social event which is the product of complex extra-individual social and historical forces. Only by understanding the construction of 'AIDS' in this way, can the more disturbing aspects of its agenda be revealed and confronted.

Notes

1 A more detailed specification of how this analysis took place can be found in Horton, M. (1987) 'Perverts, Inverts and Experts — The Cultural Production of an AIDS Research Paradigm', unpublished BSc dissertation, University College, London.

2 The symptomology of syphilis and gonorrhoea were not distinguished until the nineteenth century.

3 By the nineteenth century, such a transformation was all but complete with the popular image of woman as the archetypal syphilitic having entered the medical literature, so much so that one of the major contributors to modern dermatology, Jean Louis Alibert was able to represent all the syphilitics as women in his 1806 atlas of skin diseases (Jeanselme, E. (1908) *Histoire de la Syphilis*, Paris).

4 It should be noted, however, that public responses to venereal disease have not had a monolithic moral character. Public health and medicine have not been a homogeneous social force landscaping the same societal probity. On the contrary, conflicts and tensions within the professions have been capable of revealing unexpected insights into problems posed — for example, the disclosure of the very real fact of venereal disease and its incidence. To speak on a subject that called for silence could indicate the existence of actual sexual behaviour. Venereal disease provided evidence of the discomforting chasm between moral ideals and actual behaviours.

5 Late nineteenth and early twentieth century responses to venereal disease are pertinent because it is during this period that we can see the establishment of social complexes that still reverberate in the social structuring of sexually transmitted disease today. For example, the 1860s saw the passing of a series of Contagious Diseases Acts. These highly controversial pieces of legislation, ostensibly for the protection of troops, allowed for the detention and forcible examination of prostitutes and licentious women in garrison towns. A sustained campaign by various women's groups resulted in the appeal of these acts in 1886 (see Cartwright, F. F. (1977) *A Social History of Medicine*, London, Longman). The campaign took the form of a curious fusion between a genuine desire to protect the rights of women and a concern to defend middle class probity — the Acts themselves had revealed the discomforting reality of both prostitution and venereal disease.

6 It should be stated that our primary concern here is with an analysis of male homosexuality.

7 See for example, Tripp, C.A. (1975) *The Homosexual Matrix*, New York, McGraw Hill. Though the content of its analysis may refute the findings of earlier sexologists, its form is relentlessly compelled to follow the same logical scheme so that it begins with historical then biological considerations, then moves to the 'problem' of inversion and sex-role reversal followed by discussions of the origins of sexuality.

8 In Britain recently the passing into law of Clause 28 (as Section 28 of the 1988 Local Government Act), which makes it illegal for local authorities to 'promote' homosexuality, provides evidence of a similar antipathy.

9 A more detailed analysis of medical and scientific reports along these lines can be found in Horton, M. (1987) 'Perverts, inverts and experts — The cultural production of an AIDS research paradigm', unpublished BSc dissertation, University College, London.

10 See *Neurology* (1986) 36, p 194.

11 See *Hospital Doctor* (1986) C6, 33, p 27.

12 See *Doctor* (1986) 16, 19, p 6.

13 See *Hospital Doctor* (1986) C6, 26, p 4.

14 In this context, the presence of more than 3000 Americans at the 3rd International Conference on AIDS held in June 1988 in Stockholm is highly significant. Clearly this has consequences for the framing of the future AIDS research paradigm.

References

ADAM, B. P. (1977) 'Some continuities in out-group strategies', *GAI Saber*, 1, pp 72–7.

AGGLETON, P. J. and HOMANS, H. (1987) *Educating About AIDS — A Discussion Document for Community Physicians, Health Education Officers, Health Advisers and Others with a Responsibility for Education about AIDS*, Bristol, National Health Service Training Authority.

ALTMAN, D. (1974) *Homosexual: Oppression and Liberation*, London, Allen Lane.

BLOCH, I. (1901) *Der Ursprung der Syphilis*, Jena, Fischer.

BOSWELL, J. (1980) *Christianity, Homosexuality and Social Tolerance*, Chicago, IL, University of Chicago Press.

BRANDT, A. (1986) *No Magic Bullet*, New York, Oxford University Press.

BRAY, A. (1982) *Homosexuality in Renaissance England*, London, Gay Men's Press.

CARTWRIGHT, F. F. (1977) *A Social History of Medicine*, London, Longman.

CDC (1981) 'Pneumocystis carinii pneumonia — Los Angeles', *Morbidity and Mortality Weekly Report*, 30, pp 250–2.

DOVER, K. J. (1978) *Greek Homosexuality*, Cambridge, MA, Harvard University Press.

EVANS-PRITCHARD, E. E. (1970) 'Sexual inversion amongst the Azande', *American Anthropologist* 72, pp 1428–34.

FEYERABEND, P. (1975) *Against Method*, London, Verso.

FLECK, L. (1979) *The Genesis and Development of a Scientific Fact*, Chicago, IL, University of Chicago Press.

FOUCAULT, M. (1982) *The History of Sexuality, Volume 1*, Harmondsworth, Penguin Books.

GILMAN, S. (1987) AIDS essay, unpublished.

GOLDSTEIN, J. P. (1987) 'AIDS and race', *Village Voice*, 33, 11.

GRAY, J. P. (1986) 'Growing yams and men — An interpretation of Kimam, male ritualized homosexual behaviour', *Journal of Homosexuality* 11, 3–4, pp 55–68.

HERDT, G. (1984) *Ritualized Homosexuality in Melanesia*, Berkeley, CA, University of California Press.

JOHNSON, E. and HO, P. (1985) 'The elusive etiology — Possible causes and pathogenesis' in GONG, V. (Ed.) *Understanding AIDS*, New York, Cambridge University Press.

KRIEGER, N. (1987) *The Politics of AIDS*, Frontline, San Francisco.

MURRAY, S. O. (1984) *Social Theory, Homosexual Realities*, New York, GAI Saber.

ROSE N. (1985) *The Psychological Complex*, London, Routledge and Kegan Paul.

ROSEBURY, T. (1972) *Microbes and Morals*, New York, Viking Books.

TAYLOR, C. (1986) 'Mexican male homosexual interaction in public contexts', *Journal of Homosexuality* 11, 3–4, pp 117–36.

WEEKS, J. (1977) *Coming Out*, London, Quartet Books.

WEEKS, J. (1981) *Sex, Politics and Society*, London, Longman.

WEEKS, J. (1985) *Sexuality and its Discontents*, London, Routledge and Kegan Paul.

WHITEHEAD, H. (1981) 'The bow and the burden strap' in ORTNER, S. B. and WHITEHEAD, H. (Eds.) *Sexual Meanings*, Cambridge, Cambridge University Press.

WOODEN, W. and PARKER, J. (1982) *Men Behind Bars: Sexual Exploitation in Prison*, New York, Plenum Press.

6
Making Sense of a Precipice: Constituting Identity in an HIV Clinic

David Silverman

> . . . people like Charles had to develop a ramshackle, post-modern bravery, that had nothing in common with previous braveries except purpose: a series of bargains from a position that ruled bargains out. ('An Executor' in Mars-Jones, A. and White, E., 1987, *The Darker Proof: Stories from a Crisis*, Faber and Faber, London).

This chapter reports on an observational case-study of a clinic offering services to people with HIV infection. It identifies four styles of patient self-presentation and examines the role of 'positive thinking' in patients' responses to their condition. The data presented here suggests that in the course of their interactions with one another, patients deferred to culturally-shared moral forms whereas doctors gave a primarily clinical focus to the encounter. In their work, doctors emphasized the boundary between 'bodies' and 'minds' as well as practical matters about the organization of care. These issues are discussed within the context of boundary policing and conceptions of 'good adjustment'.

Elsewhere in this book, Weeks suggests that the responses to HIV infection in the West have passed through three phases. Between 1981 and 1983, the crisis dawned, and there was an awakening sense of anxiety and fear directed at perceived risk groups such as gay men, Haitians, and injecting drug-users. In 1984, according to Weeks, a 'moral panic' gained momentum. In the context of growing media hysteria, moral issues to do with permissiveness became condensed into a crisis by the threat of AIDS which became 'God's judgment' on an immoral world. Concurrently, and perhaps as a result of the perceived threat to the heterosexual population, this was also a time when governments responded, albeit hesitantly, by sponsoring scientific research to identify the virus. From this point onwards, there was also an emergence of self-help activity among people affected by the virus, often with dramatic effects on the incidence of infection within the communities concerned.

By 1986, Weeks identifies a move away from a 'moral panic' to 'crisis management'. Governments now perceived the depth of the crisis as well as its international context. Increasing funds were made available for medical provision, while voluntary bodies working in the area received encouragement. Despite a series of continuing struggles to redefine the nature and context of 'sex education' in schools, the UK government funded an expensive advertising campaign designed, so its proponents argued, to reduce high risk behaviour.

This is not to say that the earlier 'moral panic' disappeared totally. The debates about 'sexual morality' that took place at the 1987 Church of England Synod show that HIV infection remains a potent ground for the striking of moral attitudes. However, aspects of the present response are also administrative, being related to the provision and allocation of scarce resources. Moreover, as will be shown, to the extent that moral issues surface in the clinic discussed here, these relate to versions of 'good adjustment' by people with the virus rather than to 'victim-blaming'. In a sense then only the Ancients would appreciate the moral flavour of the encounters to be described, as patients discuss with doctors their versions of 'the good life'. Set against this classical backdrop, the actions of the doctors themselves seem distinctively modern, eschewing moral issues and emphasizing their specialized, Cartesian competences with a clear focus on bodies not minds.

The Setting

The clinic in this study was located in the Genito-Urinary Department of an inner-city hospital in Southern England. It was held weekly at the time the research was carried out to monitor the progress of HIV positive patients who were taking the drug AZT (Retrovir). Although still at an experimental stage of development, AZT seems able to slow down the rate at which the virus reproduces itself and so to prolong life. However, it also has side-effects, particularly on the blood, which seemed to peak between four and six weeks after treatment begins. Throughout this period, patients may be seen at weekly intervals. At other times, two to three weeks may elapse between appointments.

Like many (euphemistically-named) 'special clinics' which treat venereal diseases, this clinic was set apart from its host hospital and was a dingy place with 1940s 'brutal' decor — stacking chairs and benches were the main items of furniture it contained. Patients waited to be seen by one or two consultants (Dr A, a chest physician, and Dr B, a genito-urinary physician), a pharmacist (who discussed medications with the medical staff and handed patients their bottles of AZT) and an occasional medical student. After the consultation, most patients had blood taken in another room by a nurse-practitioner. Most regularly saw one of a number of counsellors who serviced HIV positive patients at the clinic.

In many ways, the clinic provided a good example of how medicine has organized itself in relation both to its knowledge of this virus, and to what Weeks calls 'wider social imperatives'. The range of staff present were a response to what was known about the virus and the treatment of its effects. The chest physician attended because the opportunistic infections associated with HIV often affect the chest. In turn, he deferred to the genito-urinary doctor about the skin conditions associated with the infection and both relied on laboratory staff to identify the presence of conditions sometimes almost unique to HIV patients. As Dr A put it in a telephone conversation with the hospital's Microbiology Department: 'You're going to have to get genned up on this. It's going to broaden your clinical practice'.

The presence of the pharmacist was interesting. Here, as in other settings, he could offer advice to doctors about the choice of drugs to treat patients. However, the use of AZT in itself seemed to demand his presence here. AZT is a very expensive drug with known side-effects which has only been released to certain hospital units. Apart from his clinical functions, the pharmacist thus served as the 'guardian of the tablets' and his presence symbolized the Health Authority's faith in the work of this particular Unit. In turn, the physicians recognized their good fortune in getting all the AZT they needed from the Authority and organized clear records and research projects to emphasize the thoroughness of their work.

As a not indirect consequence of HIV infection, genito-urinary medicine and allied medical practices have moved, almost overnight, from being 'Cinderella' specialisms to well-funded, high-status work. Millions of pounds of additional finance had suddenly been devoted to work in this speciality by a government engaged in crisis-management. Additionally, some doctors have found themselves in an unexpected spotlight, sought after by the media and newly attractive as gatekeepers for medical and social scientific research.

Between September and November 1987, a total of seven clinic sessions were observed, involving thirty-seven consultations. A total of fifteen patients were seen, many of them several times.[1] All were male with a median age in the early thirties. Access to the research setting was gained via an introduction by a nationally-known doctor working in this area whose own Unit, for the reasons suggested earlier, was reportedly 'over-researched'. The genito-urinary consultant in the clinic studied proved to be very sympathetic to social scientific research and was already involved in a study of health behaviour.

Uniquely, so far as is known, the research reported here was an observational study of HIV positive patients. No attempt was made to interview the individuals concerned. The researcher was present in the consulting room at a side-angle to both doctors and patient. Given the presumed sensitivity of the occasion, tape-recording was not attempted. Instead, detailed hand-written data was collected, using a separate sheet for each consultation. Patients' consent for the researcher's presence was obtained by Dr B before a first visit was made.

Patient Behaviour

Nearly all patients had attended the clinic for several months. Several had been in contact over a number of years and/or had had in-patient stays in the hospital to which it was attached. In consequence, the study involved 'experienced patients' who could be expected to ask 'sensible' questions and to understand medical statements with little difficulty. Similar levels of experience were noted in a study of a clinic for leukaemia patients in remission (Silverman, 1987). Patients, then, were provided with a good deal of unfiltered clinical information which they appeared to take in without difficulty. Over the course of the research, only two occasions were observed, both involving the same patient, where there was a notable lack of understanding:

Dr A: I think we'll do a smack.
Len: What's that?
Dr A: (is writing in Len's notes and seems not to have heard the question)
Dr A: Have we ever assessed your higher functions?
Len: What's that?
Dr A: Your memory and things.

Much more typical was the kind of well-informed questions asked here by Alan:

Alan:	And the blood counts and so on are holding up satisfactorily?
Dr A:	They are indeed.

and echoed in the following conversation between Charles and Dr A:

Charles:	I appreciate being seen regularly. It's 100 per cent necessary. Because looking at that blood count I think I'll go on to contract AIDS.
Dr A:	I think that's a very reasonable statement. Yes it does look like there's some distinct impression of immuno-suppression.
Charles:	(infection last year with salmonella) Could that have affected the T cells?

Infection and Identity

Dingwall (1976) has shown how people interpret their signs and symptoms within a framework of lay health knowledge, involving significant others like family, friends and neighbours. With HIV infection, support groups like *Frontliners* may be more central as a referral network. In addition, the publicity given to relevant signs and symptoms may mean that patients are much more knowledgeable than is usual with official health knowledge about their condition and its current stage.

Throughout his consultation, Charles clearly wondered about what stage the infection had reached in his case. Earlier on however, he had made it clear that this had implications for his state of mind:

Dr A:	How do you feel?
Charles:	Okay, You know the little things that crop up tend to play on my mind more than anything else (but no noticeable tiredness)
Dr A:	Have you seen Counsellor A?

Another patient explored the significance of his symptoms thus:

Dr A:	How do you feel in yourself?
Harry:	I don't feel particularly healthy (allergy, cold symptoms).

Don't know whether it's connected with being HIV positive.

(Harry is examined)

For both Charles and Harry, Dr A can validate the relation between their symptoms and the infection. Like all of the patients observed, both are involved in a social career with objective and subjective elements. Their objective careers will be determined by their symptoms and by the names attached to these by medical staff. Their subjective careers on the other hand involve their reconstituted identities at different objective career stages.

As Sontag (1979) has noted, illness is often taken as a moral or psychological metaphor. In the nineteenth century, tuberculosis, for instance, was popularly perceived as a disease which affected intelligent or poetic individuals. Today, HIV infection carries a heavy metaphorical baggage. Through the study, patients made reference to the shame that could come from others knowing that they were infected. For example, after being asked by the doctor whether he was taking his AZT capsules, Eric, who used a buzzer which rang every four hours to remind him to take the drug, commented

Eric: It's a dead giveaway. Everybody knows what you've got.

Personal as well as social anxiety was a recurrent theme throughout many of the consultations.

Dr A: Do *you* think it's anxiety?

Len: Pressures, anxiety must contribute to the pain but then I was in pain before the (pause) (very softly) virus.

Len's apparent unwillingness even to speak the name of the virus reveals a situation in which the 'moral panic' about AIDS seems to have entered into patients' own identities. In such a context, Len wanted to keep his diagnosis out of the public domain. In a later consultation, he discussed with the doctor whether his diagnosis could be kept out of the evidence that the hospital was submitting to a court about a marital dispute. This desire for secrecy had parallels in other consultations:

Eric: (explains that his social worker thinks he should be on

	sickness benefit rather than on unemployment benefit in case he is offered a job; explains what he wants stated on his certificate).
Dr B:	At some point you'll tell people it's HIV?
Eric:	Yes.
Dr B:	I'll put on it viral infection.

Dr B:	Who knows about your illness apart from you and your wife?
Alan:	My GP plus one work colleague (in case anything goes wrong). As much for the sake of other people.
Dr A:	There's a limited number of people you can tell before it gets out of hand.
Alan:	You're never sure if it's getting out of hand or how they will take it. They might run amok.

Given expected societal reactions like this, it is not surprising that in speculating whether he could have passed on the infection to his own daughter, Len failed to name the virus. The doctor too, in his reassuring reply, failed to name the infection:

Len:	I'm a bit concerned about Linda. She has lots of infections.
Dr A:	I'm sure it's not . . . (explains why not).

Presentation of Self

It is a sociological truism that medical encounters deal with a moral, as well as a purely physical, order. We see this in the 'personal' comments made about patients and their families in referral letters between doctors; it is also visible in many post-consultation comments by medical staff. In one diabetic clinic, for instance, staff regularly discussed how far they could believe their patients' accounts (Silverman, 1987). Moral matters are also to the fore in how patients present themselves to doctors. At two diabetic clinics in the same study, teenage patients were keen to emphasize that they had carried out the desired amount of testing of blood glucose, while their mothers engaged in complicated interactional work to demonstrate that they were 'responsible' but not 'naggers'.

Despite the social climate in which HIV infection is viewed and patients' stated concern about how far the illness has progressed, there was considerable variation here in how they presented themselves to the doctor. From the limited data collected, it was possible to identify four 'styles' of self-presentation: 'cool', 'anxious', 'objective' and 'theatrical'.

The 'cool' style was exemplified by Barry who had been very ill as an in-patient six months previously but who now responded in an entirely deadpan manner to the questions asked of him:

Dr A: (to Dr B) If he had a second convulsion it would not be good.
(to patient) But you're looking quite good.
Barry: Thank you.

Here, the doctor's comment was treated coolly with an air of politeness and acceptance rather than with anxiety or apparent concern. The consultation continued in this completely deadpan manner:

Dr A: Are you back at work Barry?
Barry: Yes.
Dr A: Are you coping?
Barry: Yes.
Dr A: I know you were a long time off work . . . Are they thinking of giving you the sack or anything?
Barry: Not that I've heard.
Dr B: Clearly this drug (AZT) is good for you Barry.
Dr A: I don't think you would be with us without it Barry.
(no reply from Barry)

Throughout the consultation, Barry, who looked very efficient in his business suit and executive briefcase, answered only with a 'yes' or a 'no'. His only more sustained intervention took the form of a question about which doctor he would be seeing at another hospital to which he was being referred for a skin problem. He did not reply when Dr A asked at the close of their time together 'Anything else Barry?'

Like Barry, Alan too responded in a cool, controlled way to enquiries about his health. Unlike Barry, however, he did mention some of his symptoms, but he played them down. Overall, one is reminded of the events that might take place in a GP consultation over a minor complaint:

Dr A:	Okay. how *are* you?
Alan:	I think the tedious thing is the lack of energy. Does that make sense?
Dr A:	I know the feeling well. Would you say the lack of energy is worse than before?
Alan:	(No)
Dr A:	Eating?
Alan:	Well, yes.
Dr A:	Chest?
Alan:	A little bit of a corrf.
Dr A:	Taking tablets alright?
Alan:	Yes.
	(doctors look at charts)
Alan:	The old tongue tends to be a bit yuk.
Dr A:	Well all in all you're not doing too badly.
Alan:	No (toenails are growing).

As we shall see later, 'coolness' as a social strategy by which to cope with the consequences of HIV infection was often associated with a health situation which worried the doctors treating such a patient. On the other hand, 'anxiety' was usually seen as a psychological trait, a state of mind not necessarily linked to any underlying physical problem. Some patients regularly treated the greeting they received from doctors as an occasion to display their worries:

Dr A:	How are you?
Len:	Quite shattered, quite weak (stinging nettle feeling, problem of itching). And headaches have been coming on.

At Len's next consultation:

Dr A:	How are you?
Len:	Heh. Pretty weak. Something I can't put my finger on. Not right. Don't know.

Eric exhibited a similar pattern:

Dr A:	How are you?
Eric:	Okay apart from the bad news.
Dr A:	We want to know how you feel.
Eric:	Tiredness, irritable, borderline of depression. Only thing that really worries me is that I can't plan anything.

Like Eric and Len, Fred was anything but 'cool' about his symptoms. Before the first consultation observed, he had stopped taking AZT because of adverse side effects. During the period of three weeks from which the following extracts are taken, Fred had once more been on and then off the drug:

Dr A:	How *are* you?
Fred:	Well this morning I had a terrible pain in my neck. I was sweating and restless at night. So I don't know . . .
Dr A:	How have you been getting on for the past two weeks?
Fred:	I hope you trust what I say but it's been a nightmare. I was afraid to go out (long account continues) . . .

As has been noted in several other studies (Strong, 1979; Baruch, 1982; Silverman, 1987), health-care professionals often present themselves to doctors as bundles of objective symptoms. In the extracts below taken from three different consultations, Ian, who is such a professional, constituted himself as an object of his own curious detached gaze:

Ian:	The other thing is the thrush you know (Ian puts out his tongue uninvited) I don't know whether I have to be aggressive or not.
Ian:	I was wondering whether Acyclovir in connection with the AZT might cause neutropenia . . . (describing his herpes symptoms) It was interesting. So you'd suggest it four times a day? Because normally they recommend five times a day.
Dr A:	But you know overall we remain very pleased with you.
Ian:	So am I.
Ian:	What are the criteria for AZT? Still T4s? . . . I was talking to a guy at Frontliners who said KS was the criterion.

Only two atypical patterns of response were observed throughout the period of data collection. At one point, Ian raised a personal concern: the possibility that he might be receiving a placebo rather than AZT.

Ian:	I think you have a fair few people asking if they're getting a placebo.

He was subsequently reassured by the doctor that he was not part of any controlled drug-trial and that he was actually receiving the drug. However, it is important to notice how he depersonalized his own concern by talking about what other people might be 'asking'. A few weeks later he was, once again, only too happy to talk about his own personal anxiety, this time more 'objectively'.

Dr A: How are you feeling?
Ian: More tired (. . .)
Dr A: Not been doing anything to make you more tired?
Ian: People say my activity level has increased. I've been taking this drug for herpes. I wonder if it's been related to that?

One particular patient, Ken, presented himself in a way that did not fit any of the earlier categories. He continually complained in response to the questions he was asked, but his concerns related almost always to his living problems at home rather than to his physical condition. Moreover, Ken took full advantage of the presence of observers (pharmacist, medical student and sociologist) to dramatize his account (through ploys which involved his audience, and by offering highly coloured versions of his future intentions). Extracts from one particular consultation show this vividly:

Dr A: How are you?
Ken: Not very well.
Dr A: What's the problem?
Ken: (His phone is still not connected) I've got a great big hole in the kitchen, leaks in the floor . . . The noise there's no insulation at all. So it's just not going well. I'm getting sweats. So I'm going to (named) hospital. I'll be nice and warm.
Dr A: The social workers are helping you with these problems?
Ken: Bloody useless.

Shortly after this, Ken once more transformed an enquiry about his health into a complaint against other people:

Dr A: How are you feeling physically?
Ken: Fine. The other thing was (account of doctor who didn't acknowledge him outside the hospital) He's just

a bloody quack like you. No offence. (to researcher and student) I'm a bad case by the way so don't take no notice of me.

Finally, after this coup de theatre, Ken extracted a further laugh out of the situation:

Ken: Is there any news of me going on full dose? (of AZT)
Dr A: I think that depends on the bloody blood test
Ken: (looking at his audience) Don't swear!

As we have seen, Ken's comments to his audience were interspersed with vivid accounts of his intentions should his home problems not be sorted out soon. His most dramatic statement produced complete silence on the part of the doctor who took some time to respond to the issues raised:

Ken: If not I'll have to go to Piccadilly and earn a bit of money and I won't even tell them I've got AIDS.
Dr A: (pause) Well I'm not sure we're too keen about that.

As will be seen later, the low-key nature of Dr A's response is consonant with the way the clinic was generally organized. The impression given was one of a routine, doctor-centred medical practice in which the presence of a life-threatening infection or, as here, 'deviant', media-condemned sexual practices rarely surfaced.

Positive Thinking

Support groups for people with AIDS, like the London-based *Frontliners*, encourage their members to think 'positively' about their situation. When Paul, a *Frontliners* representative, spoke at a recent conference on social aspects of AIDS, we heard examples of this kind of thinking:

Paul: Fifty years like I was are not as good as one year as I am now . . . at a loss when seeing people who are totally negative . . . keeping my energy up . . . vitamins, massage, not too many burgers . . . Just because you've got AIDS doesn't mean you're any

> different . . . I am not suffering with AIDS, I'm living with AIDS. I try to normalize my life in some respects (he plans to walk up a mountain next summer) . . . It's not necessarily the quantity of your life, it's the quality that matters.

Two of the fifteen patients I observed during the course of this study, Alan and Barry, exemplified this 'positive thinking' by remaining at work (it may be significant that both had white-collar jobs). As we have seen, Barry took it for granted that he should still be at work despite the near-fatal course of events in his life a few months earlier. Alan's approach to 'positive thinking' involved him trying to stay at work but adapting his commitment:

Dr A: How about work?

Alan: I manage quite well. I work just a few days. I try not to do too many long days. I've had, once this whole thing blew up, to become a bit (cautious). (Not running around doings things.) It's just an adjustment but I think we're getting there.

In response to these remarks, the doctors make no comment about Alan's account of 'getting there'. However, when Ian, the health-care professional, talked about returning to work on a part-time basis, this elicited an enthusiastic response:

Dr B: It's important for you to get a job (otherwise your anxiety will go up).

Dr A: (referring to an offer of part-time work) It seems a marvellous offer. If you could limit your hours. It's difficult for us to predict. We have to take an optimistic view.

Taking 'an optimistic view' is something which can still be achieved in the absence of paid employment. In the following extract, Eric showed this in comments he made about his prospective involvement in a youth club. His intentions too were applauded by each doctor:

(Dr A has just completed his closing statement: Eric is to have another blood test and 'to bash on' with the AZT.)

Eric: I just keep going.

Dr A: I know you're just one of those people and I admire you for it.
Eric: I must admit the vomiting was the first time I felt fear. I was shit scared.
Dr B: Has your tiredness gone?
Eric: (better) Yesterday I slept till twelve o'clock. I mean I hate to waste a whole day.
Dr B: (?) Yes sure.
Eric: I admit I got into a depression the other day. I couldn't see my future. I know there is a future. I'm hoping to do a bit of sport (helping kids at a youth club).

Eric's affirmation that 'there is a future' brings us back full circle to the comments Paul made when he spoke to the AIDS conference about living with AIDS. For Eric, the future is a matter of 'knowledge', whilst depression, like a sin, is something that has to be 'admitted'. The significance of the doctor's switch to safer, medical territory ('Has your tiredness gone?) when Eric admitted to having been 'shit scared' will be taken up later.

The Fine Power of Moral Forms

Only four out of fifteen patients observed talked at length about their 'positive thinking' while at the clinic, although it is possible that they may perhaps display this kind of commitment elsewhere, to counsellors or to the nurse-practitioners. However, when the occasion arose, many patients were at pains to present to doctors their respect for what they were told at the clinic and their concern that doctors should trust them. Even when they could not display 'positive thinking', they appeared to want to be seen as responsible and trustworthy individuals:

Dr A: You taking the tablets alright?
Len: Religiously . . . haven't missed any.

Even when other patients could not manage with Len's 'religious' fervour, they still reported a desire to do the right thing in their dealings with doctors. For instance, although Don mentions that he has not been taking the antibiotics prescribed by a dentist for an oral infection, he speedily insisted on his good faith:

Don: It doesn't help my immune system, it doesn't help me . . .
Dr A: But tell them when you see them.
Don: I shall. I'm (always) honest with doctors, it doesn't pay.

Such a respect for moral forms (perhaps instrumental in Don's case) was affirmed even by patients who presented as 'anxious'. We have already seen how Fred, in the course of a statement of his miserable experiences, nonetheless hoped that his listeners would 'trust' what he said. Shortly afterward, he reinforced his concern about this when he commented:

Fred: I'm sorry I don't want to give the impression I'm complaining about everything (describes further symptom).
Dr B: Why don't we wait till you see Dr X for this . . . (a one-week follow up appointment is arranged at this clinic)

Fred: I'm sorry maybe you think I'm completely mad (mentions fears of becoming demented like his friend now in hospital)

Even in the case of Ken, whose self-expression took the form of theatre, a concern for moral forms, albeit in a humorous context, was still present. We have already seen this in the asides he made — 'No offence', 'Don't take no notice of me' and 'Don't swear'. This kind of theatre worked precisely because it acknowledged the power of these moral forms. But Ken's style was not always theatrical. Even he wanted the doctors to be clear that he was behaving towards them in good faith. An illustration of this arose in the context of a doctor's statement which showed that Ken did not wait to have blood taken after his last visit:

Dr A: Only thing I want you to do is to have a blood test.
Ken: I did genuinely forget last time.
Dr A: I'm sure.

Faced with the doctor's implied moral charge, Ken's discourse switched abruptly from that of theatre to that of moral certainty. Following this transformation, Dr A seemed quite prepared to forget all that has gone before and to accept Ken's new persona — an honest man who had made a 'genuine' mistake.

Doctor Behaviour

I commented above about how Ken's outburst about earning money from prostitution was out of key with the general tenor of doctor–patient business in this clinic. On the surface, the context of the study was a routine, doctor-centred medical practice in which doctors' business was the prime focus of the exchange: patients generally acted as if the central matter at hand was the monitoring of their health (particularly their blood) in the context of taking AZT.

The *clinical* focus of these encounters was shown in a number of ways. First, they tend to involve, on average, relatively short encounters the mean length being fifteen minutes. This, together with a busy waiting room and a traditional consulting room with a doctor seated behind a desk, suggested a highly focused, clinical encounter. Second, doctors generally responded to social and psychological issues volunteered by the patient by reverting to clinical matters, except when applauding particular patient actions and/or referring the patient to a counsellor. The only other exception to this rule occurred when patients displayed 'positive thinking'. Third, doctors' only regular point of entry into the psyches of their patients was via reassurance about how well they were doing on AZT and via a commitment to 'bash on' with the treatment. Occasionally, they also appealed to patients' decision-making rights when it came to deciding about whether or not to go on the drug, as is shown in the following interchange.

Dr A:	What would you like to do.
Fred:	You know what's best.
Dr A:	No, you know.
Fred:	Well, AZT is the only answer.
Fred:	. . . maybe try it for two weeks.
Dr A:	So we'll try for another two weeks.

This kind of 'consumerism' by doctors may parallel what happens in other non life-threatening conditions where the treatment may have deleterious side-effects. Finally, doctors provided few opportunities for patients to ask questions. So patients had to create their own spaces:

Fred:	Can I have two minutes more?
Dr A:	Yes.
Fred:	(asks a series of questions)

'Bodies' not 'Minds'

We have already seen how doctors in this clinic emphasized medical matters and rarely respond to the opportunity to discuss psychological issues. This strategy is shown particularly vividly in the following interchange which took place after Eric had talked about his fear that others might be alerted to his condition via the buzzer which reminded him to take his AZT. On this occasion, the doctor did not use the opportunity provided to explore the cause of Eric's fears but returned swiftly to the clinical realm:

Eric:	It's a dead giveaway. Everybody knows what you've got . . .
Eric:	(comments on his weight — it is steady).
Dr A:	I'm glad you don't feel worse.
Eric:	(can cope; long statement about tiredness, followed by long periods of sleep).
Dr A:	Okay so we bash on . . . not expecting any problems I don't want to say anything inappropriate. But we're very encouraged by this treatment (had people far worse than you do well).

However, it did not seem that this doctor was reluctant to enter the non-clinical realm simply because of the 'negative' responses he might have to deal with. When Eric became more 'positive' about the changes in his outlook and relationships that had come with starting on AZT, Dr A responded at most minimally:

Eric:	Before I was offered all this . . . all sorts of problems. People were suggesting meditation.

(Dr A is looking down, writing Eric's blood test results into the notes; there is no eye contact)

	so I want to take it.
Dr A:	(looks up) Well that's right.
Eric:	My parents were quite worried about it (AZT-DS).

Dr A:	They must watch TV.
Eric:	Now they'll talk about it. We might even start a relationship heh heh.
Dr A:	Good (arranges next appointment).

Elsewhere, when patients volunteered statements about their 'anxieties', Dr A responded by putting them in touch with a counsellor. The following interchange came during his assessment of whether Charles who was first diagnosed two years earlier and who now had herpes and a low T4 cell count, should go on AZT:

Dr A:	How do you feel?
Charles:	Okay. You know the little things that crop up tend to play on my mind more than anything else . . .
Dr A:	Have you seen counsellor A?
Charles:	No that's tomorrow. Eleven o'clock.
Dr A:	(looks through the notes; raises with Charles whether he should now go on to AZT).

Here, Charles has interpreted Dr A's question ('How do you feel?) in relation to his state of mind. In another consultation, Harry, who is also not yet on AZT, responded in a similar way to a question about the cause of his sleeping difficulties. Once again, he was swiftly passed on to a counsellor:

Harry:	I don't know why but I don't seem to be sleeping.
Dr A:	Why do you think this is?
Harry:	Because I'm anxious about things.
Dr B:	How about seeing Counsellor A?
Dr A:	It might help you to chew over these things if we found a sympathetic psychologist. This woman's a psychologist not a psychiatrist.

Only on three deviant occasions did the focus move to 'minds' rather than 'bodies'. Barry, who has already been described as 'cool', responded throughout his consultations in a deadpan manner to the doctors' enquiries. All he volunteered when asked was that he felt a little tired. On one occasion, and out of the blue, Dr A switched from a statement about the good effects of AZT to an enquiry about Barry's home situation:

Dr A:	Anything else Barry?

Dr A: And you're more tired than you were.
Dr B: Clearly this drug is good for Barry.
Dr A: I don't think you would be with us without it Barry.
Dr A: Are your parents still with you?
Barry: No.
Dr A: All the more reason to take the drugs religiously.

Dr A's final utterance employed the same word ('religiously') that Len had used (one wonders if there is anything about this condition and the absence of a cure for it which encourages this vocabulary — or is the term used when discussing treatments for other conditions?). More relevant here was the way in which Dr A's remark transformed what might have been a 'social' enquiry into a clinical issue of compliance.

A second deviant case can be found in the consultation with Eric already discussed. Here, Dr A appeared at first to be asking about Eric's state of mind. However, Eric's response was simply used as the pretext for a further set of clinical questions and, like Charles and Harry, he was quickly referred to a counsellor to 'unravel' his mental condition:

Dr A: How are you?
Eric: Okay apart from the bad news.
Dr A: We want to know how you feel.
Eric: Tiredness, irritable, borderline of depression.
Dr A: (Questions about activity levels, appetite, mental processes) Okay. Well no doubt Counsellor A will unravel this.

In both of these cases, the move outside a clinical frame of reference was temporary. Significantly, after Eric had left the consulting room, Dr A discussed with the pharmacist present the *physical* bases of Eric's reported 'feelings' in the context of the possibility of formal exercise tests or tests for aphasia.

Only the third deviant case did not move so quickly from 'mind' to 'body'. It occurred in one of Alan's consultations when Doctor B asked, 'Who knows about your illness apart from you and your wife?' As we have already seen, this led to a discussion of the problems of telling people about your condition which did not immediately lead back into purely clinical matters.

It would be wrong to give the impression that the doctors in this clinic were wrong to focus on 'bodies' rather than on 'minds'. Indeed, in earlier work I have identified some of the difficulties and double-binds that can arise when doctors discuss patients' 'minds' and home circumstances (Silverman, 1987). There are clearly important issues at stake here that will need to be returned to later. For the moment, I want to focus on how, as in Eric's case, doctors were able to identify underlying patterns behind patients' preferred modes of self-presentation. In order to do this it is necessary to return to the typology of patients' style of self-presentation to examine the varying ways in which the doctors responded to each patient's account.

'Coolness' as a Reality and as a Problem

Earlier we saw how the doctors interpreted Barry's and Alan's apparent 'cool' styles of self-presentation in radically different ways. After Barry's consultation was over, I turned to a doctor to comment on how calm Barry had seemed:

DS:	(he seems very calm)
Dr A:	Yes he is.
DS:	Has he been counselled?
Dr A:	He's getting all the support he needs. My own view is that you can overdo the counselling.

So Dr A wanted to treat Barry's 'calm' state as a reality which required no further investigation. Conversely, Alan who was seen twenty minutes later and who appeared to show even more coolness in the efforts he made to pull the doctor's leg, was perceived very differently.

DS:	Another cool customer?
Dr A:	He's a very complex character. Difficult to sort out his sexual . . .

Unlike most of the patients seen in this clinic, Alan is married and this gave Dr A reason to treat his 'coolness' as perhaps not at all as it seems.

Such an interpretation made sense of an account that Dr B had offered of Alan after a previous appointment:

Dr B:	I don't think Alan is very well (very shaky, chronic

	pain and herpes) He's not told us about it. He's not told people about his HIV.
Dr B:	I think keep an eye on him. I think he's saying he's well but he's not.

So apparently similar behaviours can be read in very different ways. Barry's coolness is 'real', whereas Alan's is a problem. This implies no necessary illogicality on the doctor's part. In the nature of things, talk does not speak for itself and an appropriate context has to be appealed to for its underlying pattern to be revealed.

The Impenetrable Meaning of 'Anxiety'

One of the clearest findings from this study was the uniform response that apparently 'anxious' patients received: reassurance and referral to a counsellor. After the consultation terminated, however, doctors routinely speculated about what this 'anxiety' might really mean. It seemed difficult for them to sort out whether patients' reported symptoms derived from the infection, from the side-effects of AZT or perhaps from factors deep within the psyche. Post-consultation comments abut three patients indicated the doctors' sense of puzzlement in each case:

In the case of Fred, Dr A commented,

Dr A:	He's not an easy patient to assess. I think there's a lot of panic there.
Pharmacist:	(Nice to assess his fatigue)
	(Discussion of objective tests of muscle-performance)
Dr A:	He's just impossible isn't he? It's as clear as mud to me how much this related to AZT.
Pharmacist:	Well the DI (?) effects are listed. But I think on any drug . . . The placebo effect was severe on the trials.

And in the case of Len, Dr A and Dr B discussed the situation as follows:

Dr A:	I don't know why this guy's getting pain.
Dr B:	It's a mystery to me.
Dr A:	I can understand the pain people saying to me he's a nut but in most other respects he's not a (psychogenic?).

Dr B: No he seems quite a practical man.
Dr B: (Defining Len's condition).
Dr A: Difficult to say. Main problem in life has been tiredness, skin rash, chest problems.
Dr B: One of his problems is he's poly-symptomatic.
Dr A: I agree he's one of our problem patients. In terms of assessment.

Finally, in the case of Don, Dr A felt,

Dr A: (to medical student) It's very difficult to know whether this lethargy is due to the virus or to other factors (moved to definite ARC). You can talk to this guy all day but what he wants is practical help. That's why the social worker is terribly important.
Dr A: (to pharmacist) A bundle of misery. A bundle of controlled misery. One shouldn't get too depressed with these patients at times.

With 'anxious' patients like these, doctors often admitted that assessment was very difficult. As with Fred, they aimed where possible to use 'objective' tests to assess the extent to which reported symptoms were 'real'. Generally, though, they found reports of 'lethargy', 'pain', 'panic' and 'fatigue' quite impenetrable in terms of their clinical perspective.[4]

'Objective' and 'theatrical' presentations on the other hand created no such difficulties. Ian's 'objective' account of his symptoms was treated as an invitation to engage in a clinical discussion with the patient about the condition and its treatment. This intra-professional conversation subsequently became an occasion for jokes and banter. Ken's 'theatrical' presentation also encouraged this kind of response — when the doctors themselves could get a word in. Unlike Ian's consultation, however, when Ken left, his behaviour was quickly put in context:

Dr A: (to researcher): The thing about Ken is that he was very ill indeed. He had an HIV dementia, no will to go on living. Put him on to AZT and he's changed. Good to see.

The Social Organization of Care

A central issue raised by this study concerns the division of labour between staff working in the clinic. Currently, most patients see a counsellor as well as a doctor and recently, a male nurse-practitioner sees them after (and between) medical consultations to take blood. Patients frequently volunteer statements to him about their experiences and feelings. One issue that needs to be considered here is whether there should be a sharply-defined focus in each of the different contexts.

For instance, should doctors focus on 'bodies' rather than 'minds'? The present practice has a certain logic. This is what doctors are trained to do after all, and it is not clear what patients would gain if doctors were to open up social and psychological issues. Moreover, in this setting there are counsellors available specifically to handle such matters. On the other hand, is it confusing or upsetting to patients for their consultation to have the largely clinical focus that it does? Or is is this what they want, given their presumed need for reassurance in the context of a life-threatening condition which is being treated with a drug with adverse side-effects? Moreover, how far do (and should) counsellors get involved in a discussion of clinical matters with patients? Should counselling aim to be a mirror-image of the medical consultation with the emphasis on 'minds' but not 'bodies'? If so, how do patients react to this division of labour?

Moreover, how far is it worth considering making changes in the organization of care? For instance, would there be any benefit in having counsellors present at medical consultations? And would case-conferences of the whole care-team (including social workers, etc) be useful and feasible? Conversely, would patients gain by a shift to a one-to-one pattern of care? Since patients seem to 'open up' to the nurse-practitioner when seen on this basis, would it be better if the main medical consultation took place just between a patient and one doctor? Perhaps other doctors, pharmacists and other health professionals could be present at case-conferences with or without the patient?

Finally, what I called 'positive thinking' seems to be the preferred patient response. How far does this derive from culturally-determined models of 'good adjustment'? (Voysey, 1975; Baruch, 1982). Certainly, it is easier for care staff to relate to patients who respond in this way. It is also emphatically the response preferred by many patient self-help groups. How far should other models of patient response be explored? For example, what exactly is wrong with being 'negative', and are there other less aggressive versions of good adjustment? Are we all in danger of uncritically accepting what society expects of us? Must self-respect be only attainable via one, uniform, culturally-prescribed response?

Conclusions

Elsewhere Watney (1987) has noted how, in their representation of AIDS, the media have put into circulation dangerously misleading sets of ideas about those with HIV infection, individuals who are usually identified as 'AIDS carriers'. Images of contagion and plague have been at the forefront of many press reports, and people with HIV infection have been popularly identified as degenerates, actively planning to increase their numbers by stealth.[5] In contrast to these views, this study has shed light on a group of frightened, ordinary people. Indeed, a major case for concern may be that people with HIV infection may be over-influenced by shared, cultural assumptions about how a 'good adjustment' to life-threatening conditions should take place.

Just as 'living with AIDS' can become for some a set of practical routines embedded in a culture of 'adjustment', so caring for such patients can become a matter of medical routine. Contrary to popular belief, the 'AIDS clinic' is rarely a site of startling human dramas. Above all, one is struck most by the routinized, businesslike character of the encounters that take place within it. This may be because this is the only way in which professionals can carry out their work when dealing with a life-threatening condition, especially one that threatens relatively young people.[6] It certainly means that sociologists should not be tempted to forget all they have learned about health behaviour simply because HIV infection and AIDS appear at first sight to be unique. Nor, despite its appeal to policy-makers and funding agencies, should we assume that survey research alone will help us understand lay and professional responses to HIV. Indeed, if ever there was an area where frozen 'attitudes' told you very little about behaviour, it must surely be in response to AIDS.

As we have seen, one of the strategies by which professionals cope with people with HIV infection is, as we have seen by separating 'bodies' from 'minds'. Mary Douglas (1975) has noted that a common cultural response to danger or anomaly is to draw such boundaries. In a parallel way, Watney (1987) has argued that the media's reaction to public anxiety about the virus has been to police boundaries. What he refers to as 'the unconscious of AIDS commentary' is little more than an attempt to prevent identification with HIV sufferers by stressing the supposed sexual 'normality' of the majority of population at the expense of sexual diversity. Perhaps the beginnings of a critical response to the representations found in the media as well as in modern forms of health-care provision can be found in challenges to this policing of boundaries.[7]

Acknowledgement

I am grateful to the patients and medical staff who made this study possible. I also gratefully acknowledge the comments made by Gerry Stimson (Goldsmith's College) and Anssi Perakyla (University of Tampere, Finland).

Notes

1 Two patients were seen five times during this period, two were seen four times, four were seen three times and seven appeared once.
2 Given the method of recording used, the data discussed in this chapter should not be viewed as a highly accurate transcript of the consultations. In particular, the length of pauses is approximate and talk has been punctuated purely as an aid to reading. Material in brackets represents either summaries or informed guesses about what was said. The patients' real names have not been used.
3 This kind of 'positive thinking' may only be perceived as appropriate while patients are managing at home. Anssi Perakyla has suggested in personal correspondence that patients dying from leukaemia who nonetheless maintain positive thinking cause confusion among medical staff. Further research is needed here on the diversity of possible responses.
4 This recognition of patient 'anxiety' suggests that, despite the maintenance in the consultation of a mind–body split, current medical discourse is increasingly forced to constitute the patient as a 'whole person' (see Armstrong, 1984; Silverman, 1987).
5 An example of such commentary can be found in Andrew Brown's report in *The Independent* (24 November 1987) of comments made by Sir Immanuel Jakobovits: 'If it indeed transpires that there are considerable numbers of carriers, this minority may seek security in numbers by deliberately spreading the contagion in order to escape what they experience as discrimination'.
6 There are parallels here with my earlier study of processes in a leukaemia clinic (Silverman, 1987).

7 Two good places to look for such challenges can be found in the relations between voluntary organizations and medical professionals and in the way in which counselling services are being established in the NHS, and the division of labour within them between counsellors and medical staff.

References

ARMSTRONG, D. (1984) 'The patient's view', *Social Science and Medicine*, 18, 9, pp 737–44.
BARUCH, G. (1982) 'Moral tales: Interviewing parents of congenitally ill children', unpublished PhD thesis, University of London.
DINGWALL, R. (1976) *Aspects of Illness*, London, Martin Robertson.
DOUGLAS, M. (1975) *Implicit Meanings*, London, Routledge and Kegan Paul.
SILVERMAN, D. (1987) *Communication and Medical Practice: Social Relations in the Clinic*, London, Sage.
SONTAG, S. (1979) *Illness as Metaphor*, Harmondsworth, Penguin Books.
STRONG, P. M. (1979) *The Ceremonial Order of the Clinic*, London, Routledge and Kegan Paul.
VOYSEY, M. (1975) *A Constant Burden*, London, Routledge and Kegan Paul.
WATNEY, S. (1987) *Policing Desire*, London, Comedia.

7

Gay Men's Sexual Behaviour in Response to AIDS — Insights and Problems

Ray Fitzpatrick, Mary Boulton and Graham Hart

In England and Wales, gay men currently make up the largest group of diagnosed cases of AIDS and of individuals reported as HIV antibody positive. For the immediate future, therefore, they will remain an important group for any preventive strategies. An understanding of the beliefs, attitudes and other social factors that influence the sexual behaviour of gay men in response to AIDS is an essential prerequisite for the development of appropriate kinds of health education, and in this respect an impressive array of explanations has begun to emerge from behavioural research in the United States. This chapter examines the research efforts that have been made so far to understand the social processes whereby individuals have made marked changes in their lifestyles. At the same time, many research challenges remain and there are limitations and problems with many of the studies that have so far been carried out. These will need to be examined as social research into the behavioural aspects of AIDS gets under way in Britain.

It is apparent to any observer that a great deal of behavioural change has already occurred amongst gay men in this country. The evidence for this is hard to dispute, since it comes from such diverse sources. Three types of evidence in particular suggest that there has already been a substantial reduction in high risk behaviour. First, there is evidence of declining incidence rates of sexually transmitted diseases, such as gonorrhoea amongst gay men (Weller *et al.*, 1984; Gellon and Ison, 1986; Carne *et al.*, 1987). Second, there has been a recent slowing down in the rate of increase in HIV infection amongst gay and bisexual men attending one of the major London STD clinics (Carne *et al.*, 1987). Third, self-report studies of the sexual behaviour of gay men attending clinics at two different London hospitals have identified significant amounts of behavioural change (Weber *et al.*, 1986; Carne *et al.*, 1987). They indicate that concurrent with an increase in the proportion of gay men using condoms during anal sex, there have been substantial reductions in the mean number of sexual partners and in the proportion of men reporting passive anal intercourse. Findings from a regular series of interview surveys conducted in London and provincial gay clubs by the Central Office of Information (COI) are similarly encouraging. Their most recent surveys suggest there has been a further decline in the proportion of respondents reporting passive anal sex without using a condom, from 22 per cent of the sample surveyed in February 1986 to 18 per cent one year later (DHSS, 1987).

The most striking feature from all the available evidence is the extent to which patterns of sexual behaviour have altered. A major social change has clearly taken place with remarkable rapidity. Nevertheless, all of the surveys cited also indicate variability in this behavioural change. In the London clinic studies, for example, a significant minority of respondents reported that they continued to have passive anal sex without a condom, and in both clinic samples whilst the mean number of sexual partners is very low indeed, the range in number of reported partners is quite considerable. It must be remembered also that the individuals interviewed in these studies are likely to have received regular counselling about the kinds of behavioural change that might be desirable during the course of their attendance at the hospital clinic. In the COI's surveys of men in gay clubs in 1986 and 1987, similar variability can be found.

These dramatic changes in behaviour are not, of course, dissimilar from those that can be found in the United States. American studies too have reported variability in the extent to which behavioural change has taken place. Two large cohort studies of gay men whose health has been regularly monitored during hospital clinic attendance, the Multicentre AIDS Cohort Study (Kingsley *et al.*, 1987) and the San Francisco Men's Health Study (Winkelstein *et al.*, 1987) both identify small minorities of men who in 1985 reported high risk sexual behaviour. A non-clinic study of gay men in New York carried out in late 1985 showed a similar picture (Martin, 1987).

For our purposes, the most significant aspect of this American research lies in the attempts that have been made to identify the social psychological factors involved in behavioural change. It is the possible relevance of these factors that will be focused on in this chapter.

Risk

One area of obvious importance in understanding behavioural change in response to AIDS concerns individuals' perceptions of risk. Of importance here are people's assessments of their chances of developing the syndrome. Preventive strategies for many other health problems have been premised on the belief that increasing levels of perceived susceptibility to that particular problem will increase the likelihood of appropriate behavioural change. In this context, there are two important questions to be asked. What factors influence subjective perceptions of risk, and does an increased sense of risk or vulnerability increase the likelihood that the person concerned will adopt appropriate health behaviours? One of the earliest studies to examine these issues in relation to gay men and AIDS is a survey conducted by McKusick *et al.* (1985) in San Francisco in 1983. In this study, 50 per cent of a sample recruited at San Francisco bathhouses regarded themselves as less susceptible than others to AIDS. The health histories and the numbers of sexual partners reported by members of the group suggested that in terms of these indices anyway, their risks may well have been less favourable.

Siegel's (1985) report on the first wave of a longitudinal study of gay men in New York also suggested that subjective ratings of risk were unrelated to modifications in sexual behaviour. More recently, Siegel *et al.* (1987) have reported findings from a somewhat larger longitudinal study of gay men in New York. They conclude that 'when respondents' subjective ratings of the riskiness of their behaviour were compared with the objective scores, it was determined that as many as four out of every five men engaging in risky sexual behaviour may be underestimating the danger inherent in their behaviour.' From this kind of evidence, it is clear that other than objective factors enter into individuals' subjective appraisal of risk. This situation is, of course, little different from that pertaining to areas of health behaviour and risk perception such as, for example, smoking. At present, little is known about what the factors might be that influence subjective perceptions of risk in relation to AIDS. The role of other health beliefs provides one avenue of enquiry (Calnan, 1987). Denial of the virulence of the epidemic, for example, was identified in one of the earlier studies in New York as one factor that might modify gay men's individual perceptions of risk (Feldman, 1986),and there is more recent evidence to support this from McKusick's *et al.* (1987) prospective study of gay men in San Francisco. Here, it was found that denial of the virulence of AIDS was predictive of high levels of high risk sexual behaviour. Joseph *et al.* (1987b) have suggested that 'optimistic bias', a process that operates with respect to other areas of health behaviour, may be yet another factor which leads to underestimates of personal risk.

The second question identified above is whether a raised sense of risk promotes appropriate behavioural change. The most comprehensive study to date on this issue is that carried out by the Michigan group in relation tothe Multicenter AIDS Cohort Study (*ibid*). Their study reports on longitudinal medical and psychosocial data collected from over 600 gay men in Chicago. Respondents were asked to estimate both their absolute level of risk of AIDS and their level of risk relative to other gay men. When these two ratings of personal risk were combined, they found that 94 per cent of the respondents fell in the low or medium subjective risk index. Unknown to the sample at the time they were asked to make these estimates of risk, some 40 per cent had HIV antibodies. The authors then went on to explore whether risk appraisal predicted behavioural change six months later. They found positive relationships between risk perception and three measures of risk reduction (total number of partners, number of anonymous partners and number of episodes of passive anal sex). When statistical adjustments were made for background, social and demographic variables, these positive relationships were sustained or somewhat increased.

However when Joseph *et al.* statistically controlled for risky behaviour at the beginning of the survey, the relationships between perceived risk and the behavioural changes recorded six months later disappeared. Indeed, on one outcome variable, numbers of anonymous sexual partners, perception of risk became negatively associated with subsequent reduction of risky behaviour. The higher an individual's judgment of personal risk, the greater the number of reported anonymous partners. Furthermore no relationship could be found between perceptions of risk at the beginning of the study and attitudes six months later that were considered to be favourable to appropriate behavioural change. Moreover, perception of risk *was* positively and consistently related to subsequent psychological distress. The higher an individual's sense of risk, the greater their subsequent impairment of social functioning, the more their AIDS-related worries and concerns and the higher their negative affect. The authors conclude that increasing people's perceptions of risk may therefore be counter productive, since psychological distress may in the long-term reduce compliance.

Knowledge

An obvious source of explanation for discrepancies between individuals' objective risk in epidemiological terms and their subjective appraisal of risk is knowledge about AIDS. Awareness of AIDS must have played a major role in behavioural change in view of the associations that can be found between the dissemination of information about AIDS and behavioural change (Weller *et al.*, 1984). However, at the level of individual differences in behaviour, there appear to be fewer direct links, in the evidence to date.

Discrepancies between knowledge and behaviour were noted in McKusick *et al.*'s (1985) early survey of gay men in San Francisco, with there being no clear cut relationship between these two variables. However, an equally early study by Feldman (1986), looking at data collected from gay men in New York in 1982–83 (McKusick *et al.* had also collected their data in 1983) found that educational level was associated with higher levels of knowledge about AIDS and fewer sexual partners. There may have been more variability in levels of knowledge about AIDS at this time in New York compared with San Francisco, where levels of knowledge were undoubtedly already high. Other evidence suggests that for some time public concern and awareness about AIDS in New York may have lagged significantly behind San Francisco. Moreover, early in the epidemic, level of knowledge may have a stronger or clearer effect in distinguishing between those who did and those who did not alter their behaviour. However, as public education campaigns begin to disseminate information more widely and as levels of knowledge rise, the effects of these processes on individuals may become more difficult to detect. This may explain why, in those more recent studies where the relationship between knowledge and behaviour change has been directly examined at the individual level, very few significant correlations have been found (Temeshok *et al.*, 1987; Joseph *et al.*, 1987a).

A study of ninety gay men in Mississippi, for example, could find no correlations between level of knowledge and any of a number of high risk behaviours (Kelly *et al.*, 1987), but it is perhaps significant that on an AIDS knowledge test with a maximum score of 33, the mean score for the sample was almost 26. In this kind of situation, statistical relationships may also be unstable. In the impressive longitudinal study by Joseph *et al.* (1987a), the predictive effects of knowledge over a six month period were not significant, but in a report on data from a further wave in the longitudinal study, in which actual high risk behaviour was reduced from 35 per cent to only 6 per cent of the sample, level of knowledge re-emerged as a significant predictor of behavioural change (Joseph *et al.*, 1987c).

Of course, the absence of an association between knowledge and behaviour is not necessarily a discouraging finding from the point of view of health education. In all of the American surveys (McKusick *et al.*, 1985; Kotarba and Lang, 1986; Temoshok *et al.*, 1986) knowledge about AIDS is very high and gay men have been found to be considerably more knowledgeable about AIDS than heterosexual respondents (Bologne and Johnson, 1986; Temoshok *et al.*, 1987). It would therefore seem that, whilst knowledge of AIDS may be an important contextual factor influencing the behaviour of gay men, in some studies there may not be sufficient variability in levels of knowledge to produce significant effects on individual differences in behaviour. It may be that knowledge about AIDS has had its full impact in influencing behaviour; what may still be important is whether or not the individual endorses or accepts the implications of information about AIDS. This may offer some explanation for McKusick *et al.*'s (1987) research that *level of agreement* with risk reduction guidelines does predict the adoption of safer sexual behaviour.

There are no British studies that have reported associations between levels of knowledge, perceptions of risk and behavioural change, but the high levels of knowledge identified by the COI in their surveys (DHSS, 1987) suggests that patterns here may well resemble those found in the United States. In this context, it has to be remembered that knowledge *alone* is unlikely to bring about changes in sexual behaviour, and that it is unreasonable to expect there to be a simple relationship between knowledge and behavioural change.

Locus of Control

It can be argued that the effects of arousing individuals' sense of risk, and increasing their levels of knowledge may be limited if one does not also enhance the view that something can be done to avoid a serious health problem such as AIDS and that the individual is capable of taking such action. There are two components here that are important — first, the belief that the virus *can* be avoided and second, the belief that one can *personally* do something to avoid it. In this context, McKusick, Conant and Coates (1985) have distinguished between 'response efficacy', the belief that infection by HIV is avoidable, and 'personal efficacy', the belief that one's own personal capacities can play a role in avoiding infection.

Response Efficacy

With respect to the first of these considerations, there is some qualitative evidence from research carried out in Houston in 1984 to suggest that some gay men may regard AIDS as unavoidable because they believe that resistance or infection is entirely genetically determined (Kotarba and Lang, 1986). But on the whole, there are few reports in the American literature identifying fatalistic views about the likelihood of infection. Most studies report widespread belief that infection can indeed be avoided. This must be regarded as a success of health education about the virus and its modes of transmission. In Britain too, 92 per cent of gay men have recently endorsed the statement 'There are several ways to reduce the risks of catching AIDS' (DHSS, 1987). More attention has therefore to be given to the second dimension of efficacy — whether individuals feel personally able to do things to avoid infection.

Personal Efficacy

The strongest evidence to date identifying the importance of personal efficacy as a factor affecting changes in sexual behaviour has been provided by McKusick *et al.* (1987). In a long-term longitudinal behavioural investigation of two separate cohorts of gay men in San Francisco, one of which is the San Francisco Men's Health Study, they report that personal efficacy is the single most powerful factor influencing behavioural change in both samples.

It is remarkable therefore that while researchers in the Michigan part of the MultiCentre AIDS Cohort study (studying a cohort of gay men in Chicago) found that measures of individuals' sense of ability to change behaviour were strongly and significantly associated with several different behaviour changes in their cross-sectional data, when correlations with the six months follow up data were examined, these associations all disappeared (Joseph *et al.*, 1987a). Sense of personal efficacy also remained unrelated to behavioural change in their longer term two year follow up (Joseph *et al.*, 1987c). Two obvious possibilities might account for differences between these two longitudinal studies. First there may be important cultural differences between San Francisco and Chicago that influence concepts such as personal efficacy. So far, regionally derived cultural differences have received little explicit attention in this kind of behavioural research even when, as is the case with the MACS study, large numbers of gay men have been recruited from very different parts of the USA. A second equally plausible explanation would be that such differences are due to problems of measurement rather than reality.

The assumption behind most studies of locus of control-type concepts in relation to other areas of health behaviour is that individuals with a strong sense of personal efficacy or those with a high level of internal locus of control will find the adoption of recommended behavioural changes easier than those without this sense of personal control (Wallston and Wallston, 1981). However, Kotarba and Lang (1986) have suggested that a more complex set of relationships may pertain between these two sets of variables. In 1984, they carried out a qualitative study of forty-eight gay men in Houston. In analyzing their sexual behaviour, they were able to distinguish two sub-groups: those with a *public* lifestyle characterized by high levels of sexual activity with multiple and/or anonymous partners, and those with more *private* lifestyles characterized by a tendency towards monogamous or closed relationships. They found also that the two groups differed in their concern about health, with there being higher levels of concern amongst gay men in the latter of these two groups.

Those in the *private* lifestyle group, as theories of locus of control would predict, showed a strong internal locus of control. When asked about how they might avoid the risk of AIDS, they adhered to the medical model, and this was reflected in their behaviour. Those in the *public* lifestyle group, however, continued to involve themselves in high risk behaviour despite having a 'sophisticated knowledge' of AIDS. It might be predicted that members of this group would all score low on locus of control, but this did not prove to be the case. While some did indeed display the kind of fatalism that is often associated with 'external control', referring for example to genetic predisposition as a factor that made it difficult for them to change their behaviour, others felt personally that they could do a great deal to avoid AIDS, even whilst living in the fast lane. This latter group appeared to subscribe to a holistic view of health and believed that people could avoid AIDS by staying generally healthy and by concentrating on things like avoiding stress.

These kind of complex relationships make it less surprising that personal efficacy *per se* is not predictive of behavioural change. Constructs like these clearly interact with other beliefs and perceptions in bringing about changes in behaviour. In future research it may be necessary to examine highly interactive processes in order to adequately explain the circumstances under which behavioural change does and does not take place.

Social Support

One of the main influences that might be expected to have an effect on sexual behaviour change is that of social support, social pressure, and social norms. In the Michigan study of gay men in Chicago referred to earlier, active participation in gay organizations, living in gay neighbourhoods and having gay friends played no role in explaining behavioural change, either cross sectionally or in the follow-up surveys (Joseph *et al.*, 1987a, 1987b and 1987c). This result is consistent with Siegel *et al.'s* (1987) findings from a New York-based longitudinal study. In this, it was found that gay network affiliation was not predictive of behavioural change. Neither was active participation in gay organizations in the longitudinal study by McKusick *et al.* (1987). Indeed, this would appear to be one of the few consistently reported findings in the research to date. It should not, however, be taken to imply that gay organizations have had no demonstrable effect in fostering behavioural change.

Perhaps the single most powerful influence in promoting behavioural change has been the more indirect role of gay organizations in disseminating and promoting alternative values and creating new systems of normative beliefs. With regard to social norms, there is interesting evidence from the Kotarba and Lang (1986) study. In their small-scale study of gay men in Houston, the group who had stayed consistently 'private' in their lifestyles were those who lived in closed or monogamous relationships. Kotarba and Lang found that this group was characterized not only by high levels of internal control, but also by what the authors refer to as a 'moral dimension' in their views about AIDS and the gay community. They sharply distinguished between people like themselves who were perceived as behaving responsibly in relation to AIDS and others who were irresponsible. In the Michigan prospective study, beliefs about how gay men in general were changing their sexual behaviour proved to be the one really powerful and consistent predictor of changes in sexual behaviour six months later (Joseph *et al.*, 1987a) As a predictor of behavioural change, this factor remained statistically significant even in their fourth wave of questionnaires (Joseph *et al.*, 1987c). The researchers explain these findings in terms of 'normative' effects. These studies suggest the important role that gay community values and morality may play in producing behavioural change. They are of interest not only because the effects they identify are so powerful but because they provide support for the claims of those who attribute the cause of behavioural change in gay men to bodies such as gay self help groups which have attempted not only to disseminate knowledge but to alter values more generally.

Costs and Benefits

The Health Belief Model is one of the most widely used frameworks for trying to understand the social-psychological factors that influence health behavioural change (Rosenstock, 1974a and 1974b). It has been used to explain behaviour in such diverse areas as smoking (Weinberg *et al.*, 1981), attendance for blood pressure monitoring (King, 1983) and compliance with long-term medical regimes (Cummings *et al.*, 1982). Some of the American studies already referred to have also used the Health Belief Model to shed light on sexual behaviour change amongst gay men (Kotarba and Lang, 1986; Joseph *et al.*, 1987a). Many of the factors discussed so far, such as perceived risk, knowledge and social support have a key role to play in the model. In addition, it is a central tenet of the model that the individual's decision to adopt a particular health behaviour will be determined by his or her perception of costs and benefits involved in the recommended action.

Perceptions of the costs associated with changing sexual behaviour can be expected to play a crucial role in determining whether an individual will actually change. An early indication of some of the personal costs that might be involved came from the first McKusick survey carried out in late 1983 (McKusick *et al.*, 1985). In this sample of San Francisco gay men, respondents who had had three or more sexual partners in the previous month were particularly likely to agree with statements such as 'I use hot anonymous sex to relieve tension', and 'It is hard to change my sexual behaviour because being gay means doing what I want sexually'. Stronger evidence of the importance of such perceptions comes from more recent research carried out in connection with Joseph *et al.*'s (1987c) longitudinal study of gay men in Chicago. Here, it was found that those who reported difficulties controlling their sexual impulses found it hardest to reduce their high risk behaviour. This relationship has been important both cross-sectionally and in their short-term and two-year follow-up findings.

Other costs associated with safer sex guidelines have also been identified. Valdiserri *et al.* (1987) report quite low rates of condom use during anal sex in their sample of gay men in Pittsburgh. They relate this partly to the low incidence of AIDS in the city, but they also found that some gay men held negative views about condoms, suggesting that they spoilt sex or 'turned off' their partners. Understanding individuals' perceptions of costs and benefits in relation to changes in sexual behaviour would seem to be a difficult but crucial challenge facing social researchers, since this part of life may involve more immediate, intimate and salient aspects of identity than the health behaviours hitherto examined by means of the Health Belief Model.

Age

The neglect by American research of social class as a factor influencing behavioural change in this area is only a surprise when viewed from this side of the Atlantic. Although there has been little discussion of the findings, there is evidence in the United States of higher risk sexual behaviour among lower income and less well educated individuals (Richwald *et al.*, 1987). However there has also been a neglect of less problematic social variables. One of the deceptively simple background variables in any study of health behaviour is that of age and a number of conflicting observations have been made about age and readiness to modify sexual behaviour amongst gay men.

Kotarba and Lang (1986) found that ageing was an important factor influencing individuals towards a more 'private lifestyle'. Respondents reported that as they had grown older, they felt a greater need to take care of themselves and a sense of declining attractiveness. Both of these considerations appeared to promote behavioural change regardless of the effects of AIDS. In Feldman's (1986) New York study, age was found to be related to knowledge about AIDS, with older respondents knowing more about the disease, but not necessarily acting upon this knowledge. In Siegel's (1986) report on the first wave of her New York study, the longer individuals had participated in a gay lifestyle, the greater was the likelihood that they would report more sexual partners, fewer modifications in sexual behaviour and a reluctance to use condoms. She concludes that two distinct processes may account for these age differences in sexual behaviour. First, the cost of giving up aspects of one's lifestyles may be greater for those who have lived longer with that particular lifestyle. Second, younger men who have developed their gay identities during the impact of AIDS may not have adopted some of the more risky behaviours characteristic of older generations of gay men.

Once again one is struck by the contradictory findings of research in this field and of the need to address the complexity that lies behind seemingly simple variables such as age. More recent American surveys tend to support the view that the behaviour of younger rather than older gay men should be of greater concern. In McKusick *et al.*'s (1987) prospective study, younger men in San Francisco were more likely to report continued high risk behaviour. Similarly Richwald *et al.* (1987) found that 10 per cent of gay men attending bathhouses in Los Angeles reported high risk sexual behaviour, with those reporting high risk sexual behaviour being younger than those who did not. Prospective studies of HIV seroconversion also seem to indicate that those who are HIV seropositive tend to be younger than those who are HIV seronegative (Kingsley *et al.*, 1987; Doll *et al.*, 1987).

Testing

Perhaps the most controversial combination of factors that may be considered to have an effect on sexual behavioural change relate to the processes involved in pre-test counselling, having the HIV antibody test itself and learning the result of the test. Kuller and Kingsley (1986) in examining policy issues in relation to AIDS urge that the question 'whether an individual is more likely to change his behaviour if he knows his serological status . . . requires an immediate answer'. Unfortunately the question they pose is deceptively simple.

Certainly there is evidence that would appear to suggest that the experience of counselling in association with testing does encourage safer sexual behaviour. The most elaborate study to date would appear to be that conducted by Van Griensven *et al.* (1987) in Amsterdam. In a longitudinal design, they compared three groups of gay men living in Amsterdam: those tested and found antibody positive, those tested and found antibody negative and a control group who were not tested. Both groups of tested men reported greater reductions in numbers of partners compared with controls. In addition HIV positive individuals reported greater change than HIV negatives. These results suggest that testing with counselling and receiving a positive test result both have independent effects on reducing risky behaviour. Other studies lack an untested control group and simply examine the effects of test results, rather than pre-test counselling. Coates *et al.* (1987) obtained data on 560 gay men in San Francisco both before the HIV antibody test was available and after they had all received the test. When comparisons were made between those who proved to be seronegative and those who proved seropositive, no differences could be found in the incidence of high risk sexual behaviour in the immediate period before testing. Subsequently however, a higher percentage of HIV antibody positive men ceased practising unprotected anal intercourse. By way of contrast, a longitudinal study of 600 gay men in Vancouver (Willoughby *et al.*, 1987) found much larger reductions in numbers of sexual partners and much more use of condoms in passive anal sex amongst HIV seropositive men compared with HIV seronegatives.

The consequences of being found HIV antibody positive involve acute distress, with feelings of fear, anxiety, depression, loneliness and loss of control (Grimshaw, 1987; Coates *et al.*, 1987; McCusker *et al.*, 1987; Stempel *et al.*, 1987). In some cases, the news may also result in the break up of relationships (Coates *et al.*, 1987). These psychological and social changes are likely to influence sexual behaviour, but little research on their effects has so far been carried out.

Caution is therefore needed in interpreting the results of studies on the effects of testing. Although it is not clear what the real denominator is in any study, the proportion of those who seek or accept the offer of a test varies from 31 per cent of a San Francisco sample of gay men (Morin *et al.*, 1987) through to 77 per cent of gay men at a Boston health centre (McCusker *et al.*, 1987). Those who come forward for testing may also differ from those who do not. In the Multicentre AIDS Cohort Study (Lyter *et al.*, 1987), 1809 gay men were invited by mail to learn their test results. The 43 per cent who did not respond to the invitation tended to be younger, more often non-white and less well educated. Of those who did reply, 16 per cent declined the offer of the test results. They did not differ from the rest of the sample on any measured variable.

Social or other differences between those who do and those who do not have HIV-antibody test create problems when it comes to speculating about the general effects of testing on sexual behaviour. It may not be easy to generalize from the effects on those who have come forward to those who have not. Indeed it may be that some third factor is responsible for any detected effects apparently arising from testing. The decision to have the test is normally not lightly taken (Morin *et al.*, 1987), and is likely to be associated with a motivation to re-evaluate one's sexual behaviour and risk status. Pollack *et al.* (1987), on the basis of an annual national survey of 1200 French gay men, have identified a number of factors that may be responsible for both impelling someone to be tested and to adopt safer sex. These include: confidence in medical authority, past regular STD surveillance, self confidence in a gay identity and acquaintance with people with AIDS. These findings imply that some of the apparent effects of testing may be spurious and the product of third variables.

Discussion

To some extent, early research responses to AIDS appear to be characterized by many lost opportunities. It will be interesting to see whether the same thing happens as research into heterosexual behaviour becomes increasingly important. As Hart (1987) has observed, it is a matter of considerable regret that early medical and epidemiological studies of gay men and HIV infection so rarely reported on the social and demographic characteristics of their study samples, let alone the social, cultural and psychological dimensions of sexual behaviour that have now begun to receive attention. The assumption of social uniformity amongst gay men has been damaging. Even before more sophisticated behavioural research began in the United States, more biomedically oriented surveys could have begun to examine the relationships between routinely recorded variables such as age and sexual behaviour. To take one example, it is remarkable how little is known even now of variations in sexual behaviour between centres in the MACS study. It would seem vital to confront issues of cultural and social differentiation amongst gay men now that social and behavioural evidence has begun to have an impact. The fact that a concept such as 'personal efficacy' can be the most powerful predictor of readiness to change one's sexual life style in one part of the United States and yet play absolutely no role in other areas is of critical importance. The need to acknowledge the complexity and diversity of beliefs, values and behaviours amongst gay men remains urgent. Remarkable changes have occurred in sexual behaviour which seem not to be explicable in simplistic terms which equate these with increases in perceived risk and knowledge of AIDS alone.

The behavioural research associated with the Multicentre AIDS Cohort Study and the San Francisco Men's Health Study represent impressive attempts to understand the social and psychological processes involved in gay men's responses to AIDS. Large samples have been recruited and periodically followed up primarily with a view to providing prospective epidemiological data about HIV infection. The studies have also offered us an invaluable opportunity to understand by means of prospective data the social and psychological responses of gay men. The San Francisco Men's Health Study has the additional advantage of being based on a probability sample drawn from within a specific population. However, the very strengths of such studies serve also to warn us about the dangers of incautious generalization about the processes whereby sexual behaviour may change, especially when these are made to other countries or cultures. In particular, individuals recruited to the cohorts receive regular and extensive clinical and laboratory investigations that cannot be discounted in terms of their possible effects on perceptions of risk, health awareness and behavioural change. As Joseph *et al.* have noted, social context is crucial to an understanding of behavioural responses to AIDS. It is by no means clear how unique or special is the social context of regular medical monitoring in influencing perceptions, attitudes and behaviours. It is important that at least some of the social and behavioural research that is to come explores the experiences of individuals outside the scope of medical supervision.

The stability with which gay men have participated in the medical monitoring of their health in many of the studies cited has provided an unusually strong set of prospective behavioural data. Prospective information is the most convincing in identifying factors that will predict behaviour, because the problem of the direction of causality that so frequently occurs in the analysis of cross-sectional data is reduced. In cross sectional data, associations between beliefs and behaviour may be due to the effects of the latter on the former. A prospective design on the other hand can examine the effects of beliefs at one point in time on behaviour on another, and if necessary controls can be made for the effects of behaviour at the first occasion. However, as Joseph *et al.* (1987a) have argued, a prospective design *per se* may not solve all these problems. In particular, they raise the question of the most appropriate time that should be allowed for predictor variables to have effect. The effects of many variables which theoretically should, and on the basis of cross-sectional data were expected to, influence sexual behaviour, had diminished in their six-month follow up. If one leaves aside problems of measurement error, there remains the possibility that beliefs and attitudes may have their effects over a shorter time than the six months period between assessments. However, the briefer the time period between measurements, the more closely a study will resemble one with a cross-sectional design.

A more serious problem that would appear to have emerged in the Michigan study concerns the instability of key causal effects over time. Specifically, knowledge about AIDS proved to be a significant predictor in cross-sectional and two-year follow up data but not in terms of intermediate, six-month follow-up data. This could have been because, as high risk sexual behaviour continues to decline, we are explaining the behaviour of a decreasing and changing group of individuals. The dependent variable, high risk behaviour, was reported by 35 per cent of the Michigan cohort at the beginning of the study and by 6 per cent by the most recent 1986 wave. The variables that account for the adoption of innovative behaviour by one minority will not necessarily be appropriate for explaining the resistance to change of a different minority.

Understanding the factors influencing gay sexual behaviour is, in short, difficult because of the dynamic nature of possible causal variables, the social context, and the changing character of the variable to be explained. To take a simple example, variables known to have some effect in changing behaviour such as whether or not an individual knows someone with AIDS may become more frequent (Burton *et al.*, 1986; Siegel *et al.*, 1987; McKusick *et al.*, 1987). Perceptions of risk may similarly be influenced by perceptions of the incidence of infection. Perhaps in the end such dynamic factors, whilst causally important and statistically predictive, will be found to be more ephemeral in their importance than the effects of normative values and personal efficacy which have most clearly been influential in the USA over long periods of time and which have clearer policy implications. Evidence for the importance of these latter processes could have a crucial bearing on the choices to be made between alternative health education interventions we currently face in Britain (Aggleton and Homans, 1987; Homans and Aggleton, 1988).

Conclusions

Much of the attention and effort in this country to date has gone into refining our ability to monitor basic patterns of at-risk behaviour and levels of awareness about AIDS. In many ways, it is appropriate that this should be so. In order to have any grasp of present and future health and social service needs in response to AIDS, and also in order to evaluate the impact of public and other health education services, we need above all to have accurate indications of the basic changes that are taking place in high risk behaviour. Research groups in Britain such as *Project Sigma* have shown beyond any doubt how difficult the fundamental task is of measuring gay sexual behaviour (Coxon, 1986; Davies, 1987). The same problems will be encountered as research into heterosexual behaviour gains momentum. However, there is a second need at present, that will also increase as time goes on. I am referring to the needs that will be increasingly felt by a wide range of statutory and voluntary services concerned with educating, counselling and advising those who are expected to fundamentally change their sexual behaviour. Their need will increasingly be for systematic evidence regarding the social diversity of at risk groups and the social processes in terms of beliefs, attitudes and feelings that promote or inhibit changes in behaviour. Studies in the USA suggest what an enormous challenge social researchers face in providing such evidence.

References

Aggleton, P. and Homans, H. (1987) *Educating about AIDS*, Bristol: National Health Service Training Authority.

Bologne, D. and Johnson, T. (1986) 'Explanatory models for AIDS' in Feldman, D. and Johnson, T. (Eds.) *The Social Dimensions of AIDS: Methods and Theory*, New York, Praeger.

Burton, S., Burn, S., Harvey, D., Mason, M., and McKerrow, G. (1986) 'AIDS information', *Lancet*, 2, pp 1040–1.

Calnan, M. (1987) *Health and Disease*, Tavistock, London.

Carne, C., Johnson, A., Pearce, F., Smith, A., Tedder, R., Weller, I.,

LOVEDAY, C., HAWKINS, A., WILLIAMS, P. and ADLER, M. (1987) 'Prevalence of antibodies to human immunodeficiency virus, gonorrhoea rates, and changed sexual behaviour in homosexual men in London', *Lancet*, 1, pp 656–8.

COATES, T., MORIN, S. and MCKUSICK, L. (1987) 'Consequences of AIDS antibody testing among gay men', *Third International Conference on AIDS, Abstracts*, Washington, DC.

COXON, A. (1986) 'The impact of context on patterns of homosexual behaviour', paper presented to BSA Medical Sociology Group Annual Conference, York.

CUMMINGS, K., BECKER, M., KIRSCHT, J. and LEVIN, N. (1982) 'Psychosocial factors affecting adherence to medical regimens in a group of hemodialysis patients', *Med Care*, 20, pp 267–80.

DAVIES, P. (1987) 'Towards a grammar of homosexual activity', paper presented to second Social Aspects of AIDS Conference, London, reprinted in this volume as chapter 8.

DHSS (1987) *AIDS: Monitoring Response to the Public Education Campaign February 1986–February 1987*, London, HMSO.

DOLL, L., DARROW, W., O'MALLEY, P., BODECKER, T. AND JAFFE, H. (1987) 'Self reported behavioural change in homosexual men in the San Francisco City Clinic Cohort', *Third International Conference on AIDS, Abstracts*, Washington, DC.

FELDMAN, D. (1986) 'AIDS health promotion and clinically applied anthropology' in FELDMAN, D. and JOHNSON, T. (Eds.) *The Social Dimensions of AIDS: Methods and Theory*, New York, Praeger.

GELLON, M. and ISON, C. (1986) 'Declining incidence of gonorrhoea in London: A response to fear of AIDS?, *Lancet*, 2, p 920.

GRIMSHAW, J. (1987) 'Being HIV antibody positive', *British Medical Journal*, 295, pp 256–7.

HART, G. (1987) 'AIDS, homosexual men and behavioural change', paper delivered to Health Behaviour Conference, Edinburgh.

HOMANS, H. and AGGLETON, P. (1988) 'Health education, HIV infection and AIDS' in AGGLETON, P. and HOMANS, H. (Eds.) *Social Aspects of AIDS*, Lewes, Falmer Press.

JOSEPH, J., MONTGOMERY, S., EMMONS, C., KESSLER, R., OSTROW, D., WORTMAN, C., O'BRIEN, K., ELLER, M. and ESHLEMANN, S. (1987a) 'Magnitude and determinants of behavioural risk reduction: longitudinal analysis of a cohort at risk for AIDS', *Psychology and Health*, 1, pp 73–95.

JOSEPH, J., MONTGOMERY, S., EMMONS, C., KIRSCHT, J., KESSLER, R., OSTROW, D., WORTMAN, C., O'BRIEN, K., ELLER, M. and ESHLEMAN, S. (1987b) 'Perceived risk of AIDS: Assessing the behavioural and psychological consequences in a cohort of gay men', under review.

JOSEPH, J., MONTGOMERY, S., KESSLER, R., OSTROW, D., EMMONS, C. and PHAIR, J. (1987c) 'Two-year longitudinal study of behavioural risk reduction in a cohort of homosexual men', *Third International Conference on AIDS, Abstracts*, Washington, DC.

KELLY, J., LAWRENCE, J., BRASFIELD, T. and HOOD, H. (1987) 'Relationships between knowledge about AIDS risk and actual risk behaviour in a sample of homosexual men: Some implications for prevention', *Third International Conference on AIDS, Abstracts*, Washington, DC.

KING, J. (1983) 'The impact of patients' perceptions of blood pressure on attendance at screening', *Social Science and Medicine*, 16, pp 1079–92.

KINGSLEY, L., DETELS, R., KASLOW, R., POLK, F., RINALDO, C., CHMIEL, J., DETRE, K., KELSEY, S., ODAKA, N., OSTROW, D., VANRADEN, M. and VISSCHER, B. (1987) 'Risk factors for seroconversion to human immunodeficiency virus among male homosexuals', *Lancet*, 1, pp 345–8.

KOTARBA, J. and LANG, N. (1986) 'Gay lifestyle change and AIDS: Preventive health care' in FELDMAN, D. and JOHNSON, T. (Eds.) *The Social Dimensions of AIDS: Method and Theory*, New York, Praeger.

KULLER L. and KINGSLEY, L. (1986) 'The epidemic of AIDS: A failure of public health policy', *Millbank Memorial Fund Quarterly*, 64, pp 56–79.

LYTER, D., VALDISERRI, R., KINGSLEY, L., AMOROSO, W. and RINALDO, J. (1987) 'Factors influencing the decision to learn HIV antibody results in gay and bisexual men', *Third International Conference on AIDS, Abstracts*, Washington, DC.

MCCUSKER, J., ZAPKA, J., STODDARD, A., MAYER, K., AVRUNIN, J. and SALTZMAN, S. (1987) 'Determinants and effects of HIV antibody test disclosure', *Third International Conference on AIDS, Abstracts*, Washington, DC.

MCKUSICK, L., CONANT, M. and COATES, T. (1985) 'The AIDS epidemic: A model for developing intervention strategies for reducing high-risk behaviour in gay men', *Sexually Transmitted Diseases*, 12, pp 229–34.

MCKUSICK, L., HORSTMAN, W. and COATES, T. (1985) 'AIDS and sexual behaviour reported by gay men in San Francisco', *American Journal of Public Health*, 75, pp 493–6.

MCKUSICK, L., COATES, T., WILEY, J., MORIN, S. and STALL, R. (1987) 'Prevention of HIV infection among gay and bisexual men: Two longitudinal studies', *Third International Conference on AIDs, Abstracts*, Washington, DC.

MARTIN, J. (1987) 'The impact of AIDS on gay male sexual behaviour patterns in New York City', *American Journal of Public Health*, 77, pp 578–91.

MORIN, S., COATES, T., WOODS, W. and MCKUSICK, L. (1987) 'AIDS antibody testing: Who takes the test?', *Third International Conference on AIDS, Abstracts*, Washington, DC.

POLLAK, M., SCHILTZ, M. and LEJEUNE, B. (1987) 'Safer sex and acceptance of testing. Results of the nation-wide annual survey among French gay men', *Third International Conference on AIDS, Abstracts*, Washington, DC.

RICHWALD, G., KRISTAL, A., KYLE, G., MORISKY, D. and GERBER, M. (1987) 'Sexual relations in bathhouses in Los Angeles County: Implications for AIDS prevention education', *Third International Conference on AIDs, Abstracts*, Washington, DC.

ROSENSTOCK, K. (1974a) 'Historical origins of the Health Belief Model', *Health Education Monthly*, 2, pp 328–35.

ROSENSTOCK, K. (1974b) 'The Health Belief Model and preventive health behaviour', *Health Education Monthly*, 2, pp 354–65.

SIEGEL, K. (1986) 'Adoption of modifications in sexual practices among

homosexual men in New York City', unpublished manuscript.
SIEGEL, K., CHEN, J., MESAGNO, F. and CHRIST, G. (1987) 'Persistence and change in sexual behavior and perceptions of risk for AIDS among homosexual men', *Third International Conference on AIDS, Abstracts*, Washington, DC.
STEMPEL, R., MOULTON, J., KELLY, T., OSMOND, D. and MOSS, A. (1987) 'Patterns of distress following HIV antibody test notification', *Third International Conference on AIDS, Abstracts*, Washington, DC.
TEMESHOK, L., SWEET, D. and ZICH, J. (1987) 'A three city comparison of the public's knowledge and attitudes about AIDS', *Psychology and Health*, 1, pp 43–60.
VALDISERRI, R., LYTER, D., CALAHAN, C., KINGSLEY, L. and RIANLDO, C. (1987) 'Condom use in a cohort of gay and bisexual men', *Third International Conference on AIDS, Abstracts*, Washington, DC.
VAN GRIENSVEN, G., TIELMAN, R., GOUDSMIT, J., VAN DER NOORDAA, J., DE WOLF, F. and COUTINHO, R. (1987) Effect of HIVab Serodiagnosis on sexual behaviour in homosexual men in the Netherlands. *Third International Conference on AIDS, Abstracts*, Washington, D.C.
WALLSTON, K. and WALLSTON, B. (1981) 'Health locus of control scales' in LEFCOURT, H. (Ed.) *Research with the Locus of Control Construct*, New York, Academic Press.
WEBER, J., WADSWORTH, J., ROGERS, L., MOSHTAEL, O., SCOTT, K., MCMANUS T., BERRIE, E., JEFFRIES, D., HARRIS, J. and PINCHING, A. (1986) 'Three year prospective study of HTLV-III/LAV in homosexual men', *Lancet*, 1, pp 1179–82.
WEINBERGER, M., GREENE, J., MAMLIN, J. and JERIN, M. (1981) 'Health beliefs and smoking behaviour', *American Journal of Public Health*, 71, pp 1253–5.
WELLER, I., HINDLEY, D., ADLER, M. and MELDRUM, J. (1984) 'Gonorrhoea in homosexual men and media coverage of the acquired immune deficiency syndrome in London, 1982–1983', *British Medical Journal*, 289, pp 1041–2.
WILLOUGHBY, B., SCHECHTER, M., BOYKO, W., CRAIB, K., WEAVER, M. and DOUGLAS, B. (1987) Sexual Practices and Condom Use in a Cohort of Homosexual Men, *Third International Conference on AIDS, Abstracts*, Washington, D.C.
WINKELSTEIN, W., LYMAN, D., PADIAN, N., GRANT, R., SAMUEL, M., WILEY, J., ANDERSON, R., LANG, W., RIGGS, J. and LEVY, J. (1987) 'Sexual practices and risk of infection by the human immunodeficiency virus', *Journal American Medical Association*, 257, pp 321–5.

8
Some Notes on the Structure of Homosexual Acts

Peter Davies

Until a very few years ago, it was unusual for those few social scientists studying male homosexuality to make anything more than a cursory, oblique and often rather embarrassed mention of the sexual practices engaged in by the subjects of their study. Rather, attention was typically focussed on the psychological epigenesis of a homosexual orientation or the social organization of gay lifestyles. It has, therefore, been a strange experience, over the last few years, to hear in conferences throughout the world, scientists from many disciplines addressing large and growing audiences on the intricate and intimate details of male homosexual practice. For today, there are reputations to be made, grants to be obtained and academic preferment to be won by describing activities that ten years ago were the province of the academic maverick and twenty years ago the subject of criminal sanction.

Needless to say, such interest has been engendered by the advent and spread of AIDS and HIV infection. In this country, as throughout the Western world, AIDS has come to be seen predominantly, if not exclusively as a medical problem. It therefore follows that the majority of those scientists addressing conferences on the sexual practices of gay men are medics of one species or another. Social scientists have, with a few honourable exceptions, been remarkable by their absence from such debates. This is not entirely due to indifference or indolence on their parts. The history of Project SIGMA (Socio-sexual Investigations into Gay Men and AIDS) of which I am an investigator, is a murky tale of medical attempts to marginalize, or when that became impossible, to control its scope, range and effectiveness.

The Economic and Social Research Council (ESRC), which has

the major responsibility in this country for social science research has also played an ignominious role. One of our early approaches to this body, made as late as 1985, was rebuffed with the comment that AIDS was not a matter of concern to the Council. This early indifference makes current attempts by the ESRC to dictate the direction of research ironic and even risible, were the human consequences not so tragic.

This book and its predecessor (Aggleton and Homans, 1988) are among the first manifestations of attempts by social scientists to get their act together: to clarify, indeed perhaps even at this late stage to formulate their responses to the pandemic. I am concerned that this response is not confined to erudite deconstructions of the sub-texts of media commentaries on AIDS, enlightening and empowering as they may be. It is also important that the medicalization of the problem is not merely commented upon but resisted by active intervention of social scientists in those aspects of the debates, and they are legion, where their expertise is relevant. We cannot afford to take the role of Cassandra, morally satisfying though that may be. This chapter is an attempt to reclaim for social scientists the role of participant rather than that of observer.

One aspect of this medicalization is that, when studies of the sexual behaviour of gay men have been undertaken (and this is more often the case in the USA than in the UK), they have aimed to provide parameter estimates for epidemiological models that will predict the spread of HIV infection and, it is therefore assumed, the incidence of AIDS. This is, I stress, an entirely laudable aim, and one which is shared by Project SIGMA. We intend to provide such estimates, together with seroprevalence figures that rely neither on samples of gay men attending STD clinics, nor on self-selected samples from the gay community. In this chapter, however, I propose to look beyond such parameterization towards an analysis of sexual behaviour that has, potentially, major implications for our approach to HIV infection in particular and the study of sexual behaviour in general.

Both the medical and the humane priorities of such research, whatever its faults, have been to provide as quickly and as accurately as possible, information for those whose task it is to cope with the present problem of the epidemic, those who plan for the future and, it must be remembered, all of us whose lives are threatened by current, prospective or erstwhile aspects of our behaviour. Partly because of the medical–biological bias of these studies; partly because of the extreme haste with which many of them were set up and partly, it must be said, because of the distaste, ignorance and even hostility of a few researchers, findings — and indeed the health education messages derived from them — have been couched in terms of individual sexual acts and overly simple solutions. Thus, academic reports chart the decreasing incidence of anal intercourse and government sponsored advertisements extol the virtues of the condom.

It remains to be seen whether abstention from anal intercourse is a short term expediency or a long-term necessity; and although those of us who have to live with abstention as an everyday fact of life have noticed it, few researchers have yet tackled the problem that such abstention is not analogous to, say, giving up jam in one's diet — something that may be accomplished with a certain diminution of pleasure but little hardship. Rather, it is, for many, more analogous to giving up meat and adopting a vegetarian regimen: it entails a complete reassessment of one's sexual practice, sexuality and identity.

In the absence of a vaccine to protect against HIV infection, the long term success of behavioural changes in controlling the spread of HIV through homosexual contact depends on the ability of a large number of men being able to manage the change, as it were, from a meat to a vegetarian diet. Some of the health education messages which emanate from within the gay community address this problem and it is, I believe, the duty of the social scientist, as distinct from the clinician or the mere biologist, to provide, in the first place, an account of the relationships between sexual acts rather than a simple count of their incidence or prevalence. For the omission of one or a set of acts from the available repertoire disrupts the structure of the sexual encounter; and the patterning of sexual activity must change in response.

It is the aim of this chapter to provide a preliminary account (partial and rudimentary though it must be) of the structure or pattern of sexual acts, or rather, some ideas as to what that pattern may or may not be. This attempt must be preliminary for the patterning is complex. Ultimately, rather than restricting attention to the 'pattern' or 'structure' of sexual acts, we hope that in time the notion of a more formal grammar will be acknowledged and a more complex analysis, will be possible.

The Grammar of Sexual Acts

The use of the term 'grammar' is no egregious euphuistic flourish. We begin from the conviction that sexual intercourse is a form of communication. If this is so, then each episode, or, as we prefer, 'session' of sexual activity can be no random sequence of unrelated acts, but an orchestrated and motivated series of actions, invoked in response to, and in turn invoking other actions.

The notion of a grammar of sexual activity is beguiling. It suggests a lexicon or potential repertoire of sexual actions, some selection from which is made to form sequences of acts or sessions, in much the way that words are selected and put into a sequence to form a sentence. Moreover, the words of sexual activity are parsed, that is they have modalities and most importantly, their selection is indexical. Sexual activity is learned and it is obvious that there are more or less appropriate responses in sessions.

It is a neat intellectual problem then to discover the syntax which governs the selection and sequencing of sexual actions in sessions. But this is not merely an intellectual game. For example, if it turns out that anal intercourse forms a crucial part of the syntax of sexual activity, then the task of health education in identifying a replacement for this part of the repertoire or changing the shape of the structure to accommodate its omission is very different and more urgent than if it is a syntactically unimportant item.

This problem of inducing the grammar is made no easier by the problem of indexicality. Many utterances are indexical, that is their meaning depends on the circumstances in which they occur, and are difficult if not impossible to decode or understand without reference to those circumstances. Sexual activity is likewise indexical. This is true in two ways. First, the type of sexual activity engaged in by two men will differ depending on the locus of the action and second, the response to a particular act will not be uniform but determined by adventitious factors.

For this preliminary attempt at construal, therefore, a dataset that will minimize the problems of indexicality (and coincidentally, maximize accuracy of record) was created by rendering into project code (see table 8.1) the sexual activity recorded in a set of sexually explicit gay videos. The major problem of such a database is, of course, that it in no way describes sexual activity as it occurs in actuality, but rather embodies the film-maker's idea of what his audience will find stimulating. It would therefore be quite wrong to use these video films to provide a full or even partial description of homosexual or even gay sexual activity. The situations are, frankly, incredible and the scripts, where they are more than rudimentary, are toe-curlingly embarrassing. More importantly, the 'action' is at best predictable and, more often than not, extremely stereotypical.

Nevertheless, such predictability is useful for an attempt to describe the sort of patterns that might be expected in an analysis of actually occurring sexual behaviour. Such a record of actual behaviour exists in the form of sexual diaries collected by the project from large numbers of respondents. In other words, we may treat this exercise as a hypothesis generating phase, relying on the very stereotypicality of the recorded action to render clear what may be submerged in the indexical depths of a real data set.

More specifically, the database consists of the coded sequences of sexual faction from five films — chosen simply because they were available rather than for representativeness. They are all Californian in origin. The content of the five videos is relatively easy to divide into sessions. The films, especially of the less sophisticated type, tend to follow the action through, with only changes in camera angle and, less frequently, temporal cuts. The end of a session is marked musically, with a slow fade, a change of scene and/or of actors, or any combination of these. Only in the more recent, more sophisticated products does the action cut between different sets of actors. In this case, the sessions have been rendered separate. By this reckoning, there are twenty-seven sessions in the films viewed.

On Coding

Before any attempt is made to adduce structure in sexual activity, it is necessary to have a symbolic representation of such activity: a code or symbolic representation of such acts. Such a code has been developed in Project SIGMA for the convenience of those respondents who agree to keep a diary of their sexual activity. An extended form of the code is also used to keep computer records of these data.

The code devised for the use of the respondents is simple and consists of three elements, the main one of which has the central position. This is the first letter or, where there is ambiguity, the first two letters of the street term for the list of sexual behaviours given in table 8.1.

Table 8.1 A partial list of sexual activity verbs

W	Masturbation	S	Fellatio
F	Anal intercourse	VF	Vaginal intercourse
R	Oro-anal contact	FI	Fingering
WS	Lindinism	SC	Coprophilia
D	Rectal douching	TF	Inter-femoral intercourse
CP	Corporal punishment		etc.

This list is extensive but by no means comprehensive. It is also worth noting at this point, that although the lexicon was developed to record details of sexual activity between men, it is not a list of 'homosexual acts'. The same approach, if not exactly the same list can be used with minor modifications to describe heterosexual and, less easily, lesbian activities.

For the purposes of recording sexual activity from the point of view of one of the participants, as in the diary, these verbs are modulated by placing one of the letters S,P,A,M before them. These stand, respectively, for Self, Passive, Active and Mutual. (It is sometimes also necessary to invoke an H, for Him when there are more than two people involved.) Thus, the basic code consists of a two or three letter verb, for example SW (meaning self- or solo masturbation) or PS (standing for passive fellatio). The active/passive distinction always follows the grammatical sense of the street term denoted by the verb letter. It is not, therefore, isomorphic with the insertor/insertee distinction.

To this modulated verb are appended two letters which indicate whether orgasm occurred as a result of that action. The first letter records the recorder's orgasm, the second that of his partner. Sexual activity is recorded in sessions, that is to say as sequences of actions occurring with the same partner(s) at the same time. A hypothetical example of a week's sessions, is given in table 8.2.

Table 8.2 A hypothetical example of a week's sexual activity

Sun	9am P1:	PF AFO PWO
	11pm	SWO
Tue	9pm C1:	MWOO/Poppers
Thu	7pm P2:	AS PS AF/Condom PWO AWO
Fri	7am	SWO
	12pm P1:	PFO AF PWO
Sat	9am P1:	MW AF&AWO SWO
	2pm C2:	AFO/Condom AWO
	11pm P3:	(AW PW MSOO)/Poppers

P1–3 Regular partners C1–2 Casual partners

There are some problems with this approach. First, it is not always possible to sequence the actions. Activities are concurrent, or one may begin as another is continuing. In the first case, that of concurrent action, modulated verbs are connected by an ampersand. In the latter case, a more general improvement to the coding system is necessary and is under development. It is not, however, envisaged that this will be widely used by respondents in the main study since it is likely to be particularly complex. The problem of coding sexual action, not from the point of view of one of the participants but as a voyeur, is not one that often arises. It turns out to be relatively easy to adapt the project code to this end. We retain the basic verbs of our original code, that is the one or two letter codes of the basic sexual actions listed in table 8.1. By implicit convention, these are upper case letters. We then allocate to each of the actors a lower case identifier. Each sexual action is therefore encodable as a three (sometimes four) letter sequence. For example, the sequence aWb may easily be rendered as actor *a* Wanks actor *b*. By using ampersands to indicate concurrence as before, complex sequences may be recorded.

As in the diary case, the order of the actors is that indicated by the verb abbreviated into the project code. This we call the *verb grammar order* convention. It is relatively easy to render this code in *insertor-insertee order* or mf (for 'masculine'–'feminine').

Orgasm is indicated by placing a superscripted ^{o} after the actor's code letter where appropriate. Thus a^{o}Fb indicates that actor *a* came while fucking actor *b*. This example gives an opportunity to mention a convention of such films as are here considered. It is usual, when anal intercourse occurs between actors, for the insertive partner to withdraw before orgasm so that ejaculation may be witnessed — a convention which may have more to do with the excitation expected by recorded ejaculation than any other pretension to safer sex. In the codings sequence, what would strictly speaking be encoded as aFb a^{o}W is therefore always rendered as a^{o}Fb.

Making Sense of End Sequences

I shall now consider some of the structural features of this data set, beginning with those features that mark the end of sessions. Above, it was noted that ends were marked cinematically by slow fades and a change of cast. Nevertheless, it would be useful if we could discover some internal criterion or criteria that marked the end of a session. This might, when we come to consider actually occurring sessions allow us, for example, to distinguish between completed and interrupted sessions.

It is difficult to overlook the role of orgasm as an end of sexual action marker. Of the twenty-seven sessions considered, twenty-three end in the orgasm of all the actors, the remaining four with the orgasm of at least one. In *all* cases, the orgasm(s) occur(s) as a result of the last of the sequences of acts. At the risk of belabouring this point, it therefore appears to be the case that these film-makers regard the orgasm as the necessary (and probably sufficient) terminator of a sexual sequence.

If we examine in more detail the types of ending that resulted in orgasm when only two partners were involved, the following pattern emerges:

aFb^{o}		$a^{o}W$	4
aWb^{o}		$a^{o}W$	1
aFb^{o}	&	$a^{o}W$	3
aFb^{o}			3
aWb^{o}		$a^{o}W$	1
$a^{o}W$	&	$b^{o}W$	2
$a^{o}W$		$b^{o}W$	1

In ten of the fifteen sessions, anal intercourse was clearly implicated. Should this pattern be replicated in real life, then abstention from anal intercourse would remove from the repertoire that act most likely to result in orgasm.

This is emphasized if the probability of orgasm conditional on particular actions is calculated. Table 8.3 details the probability of orgasm occurring as a result of particular activities when only two actors are involved in a session and table 8.4, those which occur when more actors are involved.

Table 8.3 Probability of orgasm conditional on particular sexual acts between two actors

Action	**Probability of orgasm**	**Frequency of occurrence**
$a^{o}W$	.51	N = 41
aWb^{o}	.09	N = 11
aSb^{o}	0	N = 29
aFb^{o}	.79	N = 14

Table 8.4 Probability of orgasm conditional on particular sexual acts between three or more actors

Action	**Probability of orgasm**	**Frequency of occurrence**
$a^{o}W$	.52	N = 31
aWb^{o}	.14	N = 7
aSb^{o}	0	N = 44
aFb^{o}	.6	N = 25

It is interesting that the most frequently occurring single two-way act, fellatio, is *never* the source of orgasm, even in the aSb b^{o}W convention. Together, these two pieces of evidence suggest that anal intercourse is an important culminating act. This hypothesis makes a certain degree of intuitive sense and is given some confirmation by a preliminary, unreported examination of our respondents' diaries. The evidence further suggests that where it does occur, anal intercourse is more likely than not, to lead to ejaculation. If this hypothesis is found to be substantiated, then, clearly, the problem of finding the syntagms of anal intercourse are of primary importance.

Anything You Can Do, I Can Do Butcher

Despite widespread belief to the contrary, both amongst academics and the general public, anal intercourse is certainly not the only, nor the most frequent, nor even the most important sexual act of homosexual men. Elsewhere, my colleague Tony Coxon (1988) has demonstrated the fallacy, also commonly believed, that there are two distinct types of homosexual man: the insertor and the insertee, the active and the passive. He pointed out, on the basis of early results from the project, that substantial numbers of men take on both roles at different times. The numbers in each of the resulting three categories (exclusive insertor, exclusive insertee, both) remain unknown, at least until more detailed analysis from a larger data base is available, but we are pleased to see that the bipartition theory is disappearing, at least from the more sophisticated of the epidemiological models. It remains, however, a working hypothesis of the project that, although role-specificity in individuals is rare, between pairs of individuals it is more common and in individual sessions it is relatively common.

As a preliminary to such analysis, therefore, it is instructive to consider the grammar of role specificity. To do this, the data encoding the action of one of the films was analyzed. The film was chosen because it uses a relatively small number of actors and portrays sexual activity between a relatively large proportion of the possible combinations. This is in contrast to other films which record sexual activity between separate pairs of actors and this allows us to develop a picture of the relative role-specificity of the actors over a number of sessions and different partners.

It is convenient to consider the sexual interaction in the film as a matrix, constructed in the following way (table 8.5).

We construct a square matrix whose rows and columns represent

Figure 5: Matrix recording sexual activity between five actors

ACTORS	b	a	d	c	e	Σi.
b	W°W			SF° FI	SSRS F°S FI	10
a		W°W° WW			SRF F° FI	5
d			WW	F°F°		2
c			LR	WWW W°W°		2
e		W			WW W°	1
Σ.j	0	1	2	5	12	20 20

the actors. Thus, in this film there are five actors: the matrix has five rows and five columns. The entries in the matrix record the type of sexual activity that takes place between each pair of actors. (For the purposes of this analysis, three- and higher-way sessions are considered in terms only of the two-way interaction.) Thus, the diagonal cells record the incidence of solo acts — here confined to solo masturbation — actions done, by definition, by an actor to himself.

There are, of course, two-off diagonal cells relating to each pair of actors. Consider, for example, the cells <a,e>, that is row a, column e and <e,a>, row e, column a. The first of these cells records the activities where actor *a* was the insertive partner (S R F F° FI), the second, those activities where actor *e* was insertive (W). Clearly, there are problems when acts which do not involve insertion occur. These are of two sorts. The first takes place when, as in masturbation, the penis of one of the actors is stimulated, this is rendered as 'insertive'. On the other hand, actions where the penis is not involved, such as rimming or body-licking, present a greater problem, to which there is no *a priori* answer. In the absence of such an answer, or more data, these are recorded so that the entry <d,c> = L means simply that actor *d* licks actor *c*.

This particular style of representation is recommended for its succinctness. The leading diagonal represents activity in the S modality: actions performed to, on, or as the self. The row sums indicate the number of times that an actor was the insertive partner in a sexual activity, the column sums the number of times that he was the insertee. In the calculation of both sums the diagonal is omitted. These might, with a certain frivolity, be termed indices of relative butchness.

The first point of interest is that the rank order of the row sums is the exact reverse of the rank order of the column sums (that is to say $\Sigma i. > \Sigma j. \Leftarrow\Rightarrow \Sigma .i < \Sigma .j$). This means that it is permissible to rank order the actors in terms of their relative tendency to take the 'active' or the 'passive' role. In the figure, the rows and columns are placed in the order suggested by these indices, rather than in that of the letter codes (which records, after all, the order of appearance of the actors).

We may then consider the ratio of the row to the column sum, which is one version of the so-called 'active-passive ratio', alluded to by Coxon (1988). These are b, undefined because of the zero in the column; a = 5; d = 1; c = .4; e = .08. An active-passive ratio (apr) greater than unity implies a relative preponderance of insertive acts, one between zero and unity a relative preference for the role of insertee.

It is clear, however, that this ratio is dependent on the absolute number of activities engaged in by that individual.

Thus, actor *b* appears in twelve acts, actor *d* in six. This can be overcome by defining a normed apr. One such simple statistic is given by the ratio of the difference between the column- and the row-sums to their sum. This formulation gives a figure in the range −1 to +1, with negative ratios indicating a relative preponderance of 'passive' over 'active' and a positive one, the reverse. The ratios thus obtained for this data set are b = (10 − 0)/10 = 1; a = (5 − 1)/6 = .67, c = (2 − 2)/4 = 0; d = (2 − 5)/7 = −.43; e = (1 − 12)/13 = −.85. The basic dichotomy (ab)(cde) that this suggests is given further weight by the physical appearance, demeanour and behaviour of the actors.

It is clear from inspection that the majority of entries in the matrix appear in the upper off-diagonal triangle. In the lower triangle, there appear only three entries, two of which, dLc and dRc are, as has been noted, ambiguous in active-passive terms if only because the penis is not involved. If the matrix described a set of actions that were completely role specific, then the entries would all occur in the upper triangle. The degree to which this is not the case can be computed by expressing the number of entries that are misplaced as a proportion of the total number of entries, in this case .08 if the diagonal entries are included in the calculation; .15 if they are not.

I would recommend these last two parameters, the normed active-passive ratio and the index of role specificity, as useful tools in the analysis of male sexual behaviour that is needed as an immediate response to the problems posed by HIV infection.

Conclusions

In this chapter, I have attempted to describe two ways in which sexual activity between men can be analyzed as coherent, structured sequences of actions rather than as a simplistic count of the presence or absence of particular sexual events. While the logic that underlies those sequences is well understood by participants, in the sense that it forms part of their 'taken for granted' sexuality, it remains to be systematically analyzed as a grammar of sexual action. Grammars consist, essentially of three components: a lexicon or set of 'words'; a set of syntactic categories or 'part of speech'; and a set of syntactic rules that define a well formed sequence by the allocation of elements of the former to the latter. In this chapter, I have described the lexicon that we have developed to record sexual activity and attempted to give preliminary ideas about the form that the syntactic categories might take. That the enterprise of describing the grammar is in its infancy is quite clear.

First, the role of orgasm was examined in a discussion of end sequences of sexual activity. If the approach that I have suggested is to be useful in tackling the immediate problem, that of minimizing HIV transmission, then it is imperative that the syntactic importance of orgasm, more specifically of ejaculation, be understood. From a consideration of the hypothesis-generating data set that was used for this study, two ideas emerge. The first is the importance of ejaculation as an end marker of sessions. This is likely to be confirmed when naturally occurring sexual activity is considered. When asked to give the criteria that they consider sufficient to define a sexual session, a large proportion of men interviewed by Project SIGMA cite orgasm as their main if not their only criterion.

Second, the overall role of anal intercourse was considered. It was suggested that, quite apart from its implication as *the* high risk sexual activity between men, it plays an important structural role in producing ejaculation. If this finding is indicative of anything other than film-makers' stereotyped imaginations, then it is clear that the role of sex education for the homosexually active male is to identify and promulgate that act or sequence of acts that can best be substituted for anal intercourse, while retaining the structural integrity of sexual activity.

Finally, the vexed question of role-specificity was once again addressed. The data here considered suggests, once again, quite strongly that a dominant = insertive = 'masculine' role together with a submissive = insertee = 'feminine' role is a feature, at least of the icon of male homosexual activity that appears in these films. Measures of the role-preference of individuals and of the role-specificity of a set of interactions were suggested. It is a prime task of the analysis to be done on naturally occurring data to discover the extent of role-specificity in (a) individuals, (b) pairs of individuals (partners) and (c) sessions. This kind of information will at least give some indication whether such a preference for a particular modality of action is a psychological predisposition, the outcome of partner-specific negotiation or the adventitious result of a context-anchored interaction of mood and circumstance.

References

AGGLETON, P. and HOMANS, H. (1988) (Eds.) *Social Aspects of AIDS*, Lewes, Falmer Press.

COXON, A. (1988) 'The numbers game' in AGGLETON, P. and HOMANS, H. (Eds.) *Social Aspects of AIDS*, Lewes, Falmer Press.

9
HIV and the Injecting Drug User

Graham Hart

As part of the government's public information campaign against drug use and AIDS which ran from September 1987 to January 1988, a brutal poster was employed displaying the bloody paraphernalia associated with the injection of drugs, including a needle and syringe which, it was assumed, was contaminated with Human Immunodeficiency Virus (HIV). Users were exhorted never to share, not even once, and not to inject AIDS.

A rather different approach, encouraging drug users to employ safer injecting techniques can be seen in the work of some of the specialist voluntary and statutory agencies serving this population. Thus, an unknown artist produced a poster entitled 'The Drug Scene' which shows, in cartoon form, a Punk user called 'Hyjean' wearing a T-shirt with the message 'Clean your works', some evil-looking Dirty Works, a small bag of clearly intoxicated 'smack' and finally a one-eyed, fanged virus with jagged edges called AIDS.

Just two years before this, at the height of an HIV epidemic amongst drug users in Scotland, neither the anxiety provoking government hoarding, nor the rather light-hearted agency poster would have been seen by the public, be they injecting drug users or not. It is the aim of this chapter to provide an account of the ways in which users have come to have the high health and political profile that they currently do. In order to do this, reference will be made to the epidemiological, social and behavioural factors that have contributed to the spread of HIV infection amongst sections of this population. This will be followed by a description of some of the positive interventions which can be used to prevent the further transmission of HIV and to support those users found to be infected with the virus. These are still hotly contested issues, however, and are presented in the knowledge that there is no unanimity amongst professionals in the dependency services as to the wisdom of the strategies to be reviewed. Some of the debates that have taken place between the professionals will be referred to in the conclusion.

Epidemiology

In recent years, the monthly cumulative reports of AIDS cases in the UK which are prepared by the Communicable Disease Surveillance Centre (CDSC) have been marked by a depressing consistency. This includes the fact that of all reported cases around a half are now dead, with homosexual and bisexual men constituting the majority of cases — usually about 85 per cent of the total. Injecting drug users, on the other hand, represent a relatively small proportion of cases, usually less than 2 per cent. Even when one includes instances where drug use was implicated but not the exclusive risk factor, as is the case with bisexual or gay drug users and with some of the children of HIV antibody positive parents, one is still left with a figure of around 4 per cent. This contrasts with the situation in Europe as a whole, where 15 per cent of people with AIDS are or have been injecting drug users, and in the USA where about 17 per cent of cases have consistently been found in this population (Des Jarlais and Friedman, 1987). It is possible that these figures will rise as seroconversion rates amongst gay and bisexual men decline.

However, in many ways it is misleading to focus only on the total number of AIDS cases. AIDS is the end stage of the spectrum of HIV disease and given an incubation period of up to, and in some cases more than, five years, these British figures represent a low prevalence of HIV in the early eighties. What is far more significant for health and social services policy making are recent and present levels of HIV infection in this population.

There are now data from studies conducted throughout Europe (Scottish Home and Health Department, 1986) which indicate levels of HIV infection amongst drug users ranging from 0.7 per cent of 139 tested in Milan in 1979/81 (Ferroni *et al.*, 1985) to 76 per cent of fifty-nine tested in Bari in 1985 (Angarano *et al.*, 1985). This last study is particularly instructive in terms of the speed at which the infection can spread amongst users; in 1980 only 4 per cent of sera collected and tested from Bari indicated antibodies to HIV whereas by 1985 this had risen to 76 per cent of sera tested.

There are fewer UK studies available, but those that have been published have shown a similar range of prevalence, with 0.7 per cent of users tested in South London in May 1986 having antibodies (Webb *et al.*, 1987) but 65 per cent of users in Edinburgh (Brettle *et al.*, 1986) being antibody positive by March 1986. Again, one of the Scottish studies (Robertson *et al.*, 1986) indicates the speed at which HIV can take hold in this population, with infection first being identified in Edinburgh in 1983, but being endemic by 1985. In the South London study cited, there was a nine-fold increase in seropositivity over a year. This reinforces the need to avoid complacency when considering the spread of HIV disease amongst injecting drug users.

Because the CDSC collects data on HIV-antibody testing test results as well as on AIDS, it is possible to compare the geographical distribution of positive test results with the distribution of AIDS cases. By September 1987, whereas most cases of AIDS (75 per cent) came from the four Thames health regions, and only 3 per cent from Scotland, of the total number of HIV positive persons, 54 per cent were to be found in the Thames region and 18 per cent in Scotland. When expressed in terms of rates per 100,000 total population however, the Thames region remains the worst affected by HIV infection with a figure of thirty per 100,000 but Scotland follows closely (at twenty-six per 100,000); the majority of Scottish cases have injecting drug use as their primary risk factor. Seropositivity amongst drug users throughout the UK continues to rise, both absolutely and relative to other groups at risk (CDR, 1988). Why has HIV infection affected this population so dramatically, and how can identifiable geographical differences be explained?

Social and Behavioural Aspects of Transmission

Although some injecting drug users have undoubtedly contracted HIV infection through sexual contact, and this number may increase with time, there is now unequivocal evidence (Friedland *et al.*, 1985; Brettle, 1986; Robertson *et al.*, 1986) connecting the practice of sharing needles and syringes ('works') with blood-borne viral infections such as HIV and hepatitis B. Needle-sharing occurs either with the drug users' full knowledge, as when two or more people share equipment on the same occasion without sterilization between use, or in situations where there may be some uncertainty as to the sterility of equipment. This occurs when 'works' are made available, perhaps at a dealer's house, and used by different people over time. Why needle-sharing takes place at all is explored more fully by Power's chapter in this book, but there is evidence from a pre-AIDS American study (Howard and Borges, 1970) that needle-sharing may take place for social reasons. That is, the activity may serve to bond a number of individuals together in a group, the prime aim of which is to enjoy the collective experience of drug-taking. However, a more prosaic explanation for needle-sharing is the simple fact of unavailability. If access to syringes is restricted but heroin (at a price) is readily available, then injecting drug users will (be forced to) use and reuse the equipment at hand. Apart from effectively transmitting life-threatening viral infections, such behaviour also encourages other physical morbidity amongst users, including abscesses, septicaemia and endocarditis.

In many cities such as Edinburgh where severe restrictions have been placed on the sale of needles and syringes, and indeed the confiscation of these when found by the police, this has led to the development of so-called 'shooting galleries'. These are places where users can inject ('shoot up') on the premises (often a dealer's house) and then after a 'fix' (successful injection) immediately leave. The practice of 'flushing', that is drawing blood into the syringe in order to flush out residual drops of heroin, also encourages the transmission of blood-borne infections. An occasional rinse of the equipment with tap water does not constitute a means of sterilization under any, but particularly these, circumstances.

It is possible to explain differences in seroprevalence between cities in the United Kingdom partly by reference to the social context of needle availability. In Liverpool, where the police have supported a needle-exchange scheme since its inception in October 1986, there is a policy of not confiscating needles and syringes; indeed on those occasions when syringes have been removed, users have been provided with credit slips to enable them to get replacement equipment on the occasion of their next visit to the needle-exchange. It can reasonably be argued that this has encouraged the low incidence of HIV seropositivity amongst injecting drug users in that city (Marks and Parry, 1987). In Glasgow, where police have not pursued an aggressive policy against small scale users (as opposed to those involved in the trafficking of drugs), and there has not been routine confiscation of 'works', seroprevalence is significantly lower than in Edinburgh, just forty-five miles away (Robertson *et al.*, 1986). Low rates of HIV infection amongst injecting drug users in London (Jesson *et al*, 1985) are again, partly explicable in terms of the willingness of a limited number of chemists well-known to users to sell needles and syringes, particularly in recent years.

The attitudes of the police and of pharmacists are not the only cultural forces influencing seroprevalence. Differences between Edinburgh and London may also be explained in terms of sub-cultural differences between injecting drug users in the two cities. In Edinburgh, users constitute a fairly homogenous population of young, white working-class and unemployed people, living on large council estates associated with multiple deprivation. If particular practices, such as needle-sharing due to unavailability, become acceptable, there is a large constituency of possible participants in that behaviour. The London drug scene, on the other hand, is more fragmented and diverse, with a heterogeneity in terms of age, background, employment, housing situation and ethnicity which is reflected in a range of routes of administration, drugs of choice and, for those who inject, needle use. This is not to say that the sharing of equipment does not occur, only that there may be fewer opportunities for blood-borne viral infections to spread through the drug-using population of the city.

Nevertheless, given earlier statements in relation to the rate at which HIV can become endemic and on the consequent need to avoid complacency, a number of services have been introduced, the aims of which are to prevent further infection and to offer improved health care to those who are or may be infected. These include health outreach services, needle-exchange programmes and health improvement teams. All of these services can be provided by voluntary or statutory agencies, although those described here are offered by a health authority serving North and Central London.

Health Outreach Work

In the United States where, in many states, it is a criminal offence to sell the paraphernalia of drug use and where the possession of equipment can also lead to arrest, the response of many drug workers has been to accept that needle-sharing will occur as a result of legal sanction. They see it as their role to encourage and facilitate *safe* needle use either by providing information on quick and easy sterilizing techniques, such as the use of pure alcohol to clean 'works' and/or by providing the means of sterilization itself in the form of pocket-size bleach containers, with directions for their use. Many of these schemes employ health outreach workers — people whose task it is to make contact with injecting drug users 'on the street', many of whom are not in routine contact with dependency services but who may be significantly at risk of infection. The main aims of this kind of health outreach work are to provide health education about HIV and its modes of transmission and, where services are available, to put users in contact with local agencies.

Research from the United States indicates that health outreach schemes can be very effective in educating injecting drug users about HIV transmission, particularly when ex-addict workers are employed. One scheme in New Jersey employing such workers to distribute serially numbered coupons to users redeemable for a free out-patient detoxification, found that of 970 coupons handed out, 837 (86 per cent) were redeemed, and 95 per cent of these people received at least one hour of health education about AIDS and HIV (Jackson and Rotkeiwicz, 1987). The extent to which this ultimately results in a fall in the incidence of HIV amongst the population has yet to be determined.

Bloomsbury Health Authority, which serves North and Central London, an area with the highest concentration of parenteral drug users in the capital, has set up Central London Action on Street Health (CLASH). This was done in conjunction with voluntary agencies concerned about the health needs of a group of loosely organized, socially marginalized and high risk injecting drug users in the city; the three workers now working on this scheme are funded by the Health Authority. Part of the CLASH workers' remit is to provide health education on HIV and AIDS to people who do not necessarily perceive their drug use as problematic and who may therefore have little contact with voluntary or statutory drug agencies. Some may be on the margins of a drug-using culture, perhaps occasionally smoking or sniffing heroin, and are at risk of being introduced to the administration of their drug choice by injection. Others may use prostitution as a means of funding a recognized dependency and thereby run a dual risk of HIV infection. All of these people are being targeted by the health outreach workers, not only with information on risk-reduction but also with referrals to health and counselling services appropriate to their particular needs. This includes testing for HIV and Hepatitis B infection and sexually transmitted diseases, access to a needle-exchange scheme and to local and voluntary and statutory agencies specifically concerned with aspects of drug use, housing and welfare benefits for young people.

Whilst such an approach offers new and potentially rewarding means of contacting some drug users at risk, particularly the very volatile group described here, it cannot be expected that this strategy alone will be sufficient to generate and sustain risk-reducing behaviour amongst all injecting drug users. Health outreach workers must be supported by a range of clinical, counselling and social services suited to the client group's particular requirements if there is to be any success in identifying and providing for this population, a point taken up in the chapter by Mulleady, Hart and Aggleton in this book.

Needle Exchange

One of the few needle-exchanges that has been running for any length of time is to be found in Amsterdam. Sadly, evidence of positive or negative outcomes from the scheme is extremely limited. In 1986 350,000 needles were exchanged and there has also been a doubling of users seeking treatment over the last six years, although it is not demonstrated unequivocally that this is a direct function of the provision of needle-exchange. However, the absence of one particular negative outcome is certainly encouraging; fears about a possible increase in needle-stick injuries amongst members of the public as a result of the increased availability of injecting equipment have proved to be unfounded. Nevertheless, there is no clear evidence with regard to the final arbiter of the effectiveness of needle exchange, namely a major reduction in the incidence of new cases of HIV infection amongst users attending the scheme.

In the UK, the Department of Health has nominated fifteen needle and syringe-exchange schemes in Scotland, England and Wales to participate in a national study of the effectiveness of this kind of intervention undertaken by Stimson and the Monitoring Research Group of which he is Director. Preliminary findings from this evaluation are described elsewhere in this book (Chapter 11).

One such exchange scheme is based in Bloomsbury on Middlesex Hospital premises. It has its own shop front, and has over 200 regular attenders (Woodward, personal communication). It is staffed by two drugs and health workers and several volunteers from local non-statutory drugs agencies. Clients of the scheme, apart from being supplied with sterile injecting equipment, are offered practical health advice on harm minimization techniques in relation to injecting;

primary health care is also available — abscesses and wounds for example can be dressed on the premises. Condoms are provided, as is advice on safer sex; leaflets and posters on notice-boards also encourage the adoption of safer sexual practices.

Some drug users attending this scheme may wish to discuss their dependency problem and the kind of treatment services available locally. This the workers frequently do, putting users in contact with other agencies or making referrals to local doctors willing to provide treatment. One evening a week, a 'well woman' clinic is offered to female injecting drug users, and on other afternoons there is an open surgery to which people can bring their immediate physical problems. It is also intended that HIV counselling and testing should be offered, but this needs to be supported not only by long-term clinical and psychological services but also a flexible prescribing policy in relation to heroin substitutes. Ideally housing and social service provision should also be available, but overstretched inner-city services often find it difficult to cope with the additional problems associated with injecting drug use.

In addition to its participation in the national evaluation the Middlesex scheme has received funding from AVERT for local monitoring and evaluation. Apart from measuring behavioural and attitudinal change amongst drug users, this study will also monitor the take-up of referrals to other specialist drug agencies. It will also use indicators of HIV antibody status at three monthly intervals to determine the extent to which the scheme is proving effective in its ultimate goal of preventing the further transmission of HIV.

Health Improvement Team

The HIV-related services for injecting drug users described so far, although within the statutory sector, are more usually provided by voluntary agencies offering alternatives to NHS treatment programmes. Many of these agencies have given priority to reaching drug users who do not necessarily perceive themselves as having a dependency problem. Health outreach work and street-based easily accessible facilities have been almost the exclusive prerogative of the non-statutory sector until recently. These strategies have proved successful in terms of gaining access to injecting drug users who would not normally present themselves to the statutory dependency services. However, injecting drug users who do present themselves for treatment should also be offered HIV-related services, and Health Improvement Teams can play a role here.

In an attempt to demedicalize drug dependency and in an effort to emphasize its psychological and social origins, many drug dependency units have eschewed physical health care, considering this to be the prerogative of the injecting drug users' GP or, depending on the circumstances, specialist hospital departments. With the advent of HIV, however, has come a realization that a more comprehensive service should be offered, and at University College Hospital Drug Dependency Clinic, a Health Improvement Team (HIT) has been introduced. This consists of a doctor, two nurses and a psychologist who can be seen by any injecting drug user who comes to the unit regardless of whether they are subsequently accepted by the Drug Dependency Unit for treatment. They receive testing for Hepatitis B infection as well as for skin and systemic disease. Advice is also given on contraception, pregnancy and nutrition. There are also opportunities for counselling and testing in relation to HIV, although the health assessment offered is not predicated upon the person deciding to have a test. For those found to be HIV antibody positive, there is the option of three-monthly follow-up of their health status. The long-term clinical care of patients is jointly arranged by the Health Improvement Team and staff at the Middlesex Hospital. Psychological support, on both an individual and group basis, is a key aspect of this provision. Many injecting drug users participate only occasionally in a drug-using culture and may not necessarily be in a situation where they can gain reassurance and advice from other drug users. The provision of psychological support is therefore essential in these circumstances.

One of the functions of the Health Improvement Team is to provide health education about HIV and its transmission to all the injecting drug users with whom the team has contact, and to encourage harm minimization techniques. It is intended that in time the Health Improvement Team will work on a peripatetic basis, and provide a service to agencies other than the Drug Dependency Unit.

Conclusion

The appearance of AIDS amongst injecting drug users has resulted in a sudden increase in medical, media and political interest in this particular population. Concerned about injecting drug users acting as a source of infection within the heterosexual population, the government in particular has acceded to a philosophy which emphasizes harm and risk-reduction strategies, rather than the politically more acceptable but practically more difficult goal of total abstinence. This has led to a great deal of heated debate within and between drug treatment agencies, as well as amongst drug workers, as to the kind of services they should be offering to users. HIV has provided the fire for these debates.

Arguments focus on two broad areas. First, there is the issue of overall treatment policy, particularly in relation to prescribing. On the one hand there is a view that users should be offered not only free needles and syringes but also, under certain circumstances, injectable drugs including heroin. Those who would provide injectable drug are often as concerned to undercut the illicit heroin trade as to combat the spread of HIV. Some who would not go this far would yet still argue for the more liberal provision of oral methadone to a wider range of drug users than presently receive this treatment. If injecting drug users were to be offered oral methadone, it is argued, they would have less recourse to street drugs and would not inject; thus they would not be putting themselves and others at risk of HIV. The weakness in this argument centres on the fact that many drug users continue to inject even when receiving oral methadone, although they may do so less frequently than previously. However, the frequency of injecting tends to rise as methadone is reduced in dose, and so longer term prescribing of the same dose may be indicated.

Such strategies are opposed by those who do not wish to see the provision of free needles and syringes, and certainly do not under any circumstances want to see a more liberal prescribing policy. To provide needles and syringes, it is argued, is to facilitate the abuse of illicit and dangerous drugs; it should be the aim of the dependency services to help people end their drug use, not encourage it by providing the wherewithal for the administration of street drugs. In relation to more liberal prescribing policy, the only result of this will be a mass of doctor maintained — and perhaps even doctor induced — addicts, many of whom would otherwise have ended their dependency by their own efforts and/or with the help and support of professional drug workers. According to this view, HIV should be used as further encouragement to stop injecting, as one more reason not to use drugs.

Unfortunately, these arguments tend to ignore the fact that only a tiny proportion of injecting drug users are and can be seen by the dependency services, even if they wish to receive treatment. This last point is crucial; many injecting drug users do not wish to receive treatment and are going to continue to inject. With this brutal reality in mind, the practical response has been to ensure that when injection takes place, it is done safely.

A second area of argument to be found concerns the strategy that might best be used to reach a larger proportion of injecting drug users than the small minority who diligently present themselves for treatment at Drug Dependency Units. It is argued that community-based services which target groups at risk — both of further problematic drug use and of HIV infection — are likely to be more effective in their work than the ostensibly hidebound, statutory treatment agencies. By moving out into the communities where drug users are to be found, and by using Health Outreach Workers, many more people at risk will receive help and advice than at present. The opposing view sees the role of drug dependency services as helping those who wish to be helped, and therefore come forward for treatment; it is not necessary to seek out new clients when in some cases there are already long waiting lists for present services.

Characterizing arguments in this way is to present views which are deliberately polarized, although to people outside the drugs field the views presented are not necessarily mutually exclusive. AIDS often serves to bring out strongly held views, and people often use AIDS as a vehicle for their own ideological ends. The drugs field is no different in this respect from any other area affected by HIV infection and AIDS. Peoples' attachment to one set of views rather than another derives from their professional location and working philosophy and although for some, AIDS has provided opportunities for new directions and initiatives, for others it has merely reinforced strongly held beliefs about dependency and how injecting drug users should be treated.

As the arguments go on, however, interventions and services such as needle-exchange schemes, health outreach work and health improvement teams are being provided, or are being planned and set up. Potentially, such services could have positive health benefits for drug users above and beyond their immediate value in relation to HIV. If monitoring and evaluation of these services is able to confirm, for example, a reduction in the incidence of abscesses and septicaemia amongst drug users attending needle exchange schemes, or an increased knowledge of harm-minimization techniques amongst those people seen by Health Outreach Workers, then these are positive outcomes which are worth encouraging beyond the present health crisis. Such hopes can, however, reasonably be dismissed as naive, or at best optimistic. Nevertheless, if these initiatives can be shown to have long-term effects on the health of injecting drug users, strategies which can ensure their continued funding and support should be pursued with vigour.

References

ANGARANO, G., PASTORE, G., MONNO, L. *et al.* (1985) 'Rapid spread of HTLV-III infection among drug addicts in Italy', *Lancet*, ii,p 1302.

BRETTLE, R.P. (1986) 'Epidemic of AIDS-related virus infection among intravenous drug abusers', *British Medical Journal*, 292, p 1671.

BRETTLE, R.P., DAVIDSON, J., DAVIDSON, S.J. *et al.* (1986) 'HTLV-III antibodies in an Edinburgh Clinic', *Lancet*, i, p 1099.

BUNING, E.C. (1987) 'Prevention policy on AIDS among drug addicts in Amsterdam', poster presented at the Third International Conference on AIDS, Washington, DC.

COMMUNICABLE DISEASE REPORT (1988) *Human Immunodeficiency Virus Infection in the United Kingdom: 1*, London, Communicable Disease Surveillance Centre, January.

DES JARLAIS, D.C. and FRIEDMAN, S.R. (1987) 'HIV infection among intravenous drug users: Epidemiology and risk reduction', *AIDS*, 1, pp 67–76.

FERRONI, P., GEROLDI, D., GALLI, C. *et al.* (1985) 'HTLV-III antibody among Italian drug addicts', *Lancet*, ii, p 52.

FRIEDLAND, G.H., HARRIS, C., BUTKUR-SMALL, C. *et al.* (1985) 'Intravenous drug abusers and the Acquired Immunodeficiency Syndrome (AIDS)', *Arch. Intern. Med.*, 145, pp 1413–7.

HOWARD, J. and BORGES, P. (1970) 'Needle-sharing in the Haight: Some social and psychological functions', *Journal of Health and Social Behaviour*, 11, pp 220–30.

JACKSON, J. and ROTKIEWICZ, L. (1987) 'A coupon programme: AIDS education and drug treatment', paper presented at the Third International Conference on AIDS, Washington, DC.

JESSON, W. J., THORP, R. W., MORTIMER, P. P. and OATES, J. K. (1986) 'Prevalance of anti-HTLV-III in UK risk groups 1984/85', *Lancet*, i, p 155.

MARKS, J. and PARRY, A. (1987) 'Syringe-exchange programme for drug addicts', *Lancet*, i, pp 691–92.

MORTIMER, P. P., VANDERVELDE, E. M., JESSON, W. J. *et al.* (1985) 'Epidemic of AIDS-related virus (HTLV-III/LAV) infection among intravenous drug abusers', *Lancet*, ii, pp 449–50.

ROBERTSON, J. R., BUCKNALL, A. B. V., WELSBY, P. D. *et al.* (1986a) 'Epidemic of AIDS-related virus (HTLV-III/LAV) infection among intravenous drug abusers', *British Medical Journal*, 292, pp 527–30.

ROBERTSON, J. R., BUCKNALL, A. B. V., WELSBY, P. D. *et al.* (1986b) 'Regional variations in HIV antibody seropositivity in British intravenous drug users', *Lancet*, ii, pp 1435–6.

SCOTTISH HOME AND HEALTH DEPARTMENT (1986) *HIV in Scotland: Report of the Scottish Committee on HIV Infection and Intravenous Drug Misuse*, Edinburgh, SHHD.

WEBB, G., BURGESS, M., SUTHERLAND, S. *et al.* (1987) 'Prevalence of HIV among the injectable drug using population in South London and factors influencing its spread', poster presented at the Third International Conference on AIDS, Washington, DC.

10 Methods of Drug Use: Injecting and Sharing

Robert Power

There is no danger of HIV infection from merely consuming illicit drugs. It is the associated behaviour, the way in which they are administered, that distinguishes certain drug users from others in terms of risk of HIV infection. There are a variety of reasons why individuals choose to inject drugs, and these will be explored in this chapter. Even so, injecting with sterile needles and syringes is not in itself a high risk behaviour. It is the use of unsterile injecting equipment and the sharing of needles with others who may themselves have come into contact with someone with HIV infection, that constitutes high risk behaviour. It is because of this potential that those who inject drugs have been singled out for particular concern, not least in terms of the emphasis of the UK government's recent media campaign and the decision to introduce a number of pilot needle-exchange schemes. All this has, to a certain extent, turned the drugs field on its head. Some workers, dedicated to coaching their clients to abstinence, have had to rethink the paradigms within which they operate and to incorporate notions of harm minimization and risk reduction. Similarly, some drug clinics have had to swallow hard and prescribe oral methadone to injecting drug users who they suspect are en route to the needle-exchange scheme around the corner. To many drug users, these schemes have facilitated the elimination of one extra problem from their stressful lifestyle: the search for clean equipment with which to inject. Most spend their time on a spiralling treadmill of getting the money together for their habit, scurrying round in pursuit of the drugs themselves, and finally consuming the chosen substances. Obtaining clean injecting equipment is often given a low priority in many drug users' day. Without pre-empting my own argument, suffice it to say that the question of availability of sterile needles and syringes is a key issue in determining the proclivity towards the sharing of injecting equipment, and is one that needs to be closely considered in light of the desirable aim of risk reduction.

Between October 1985 and October 1988, along with my colleagues on the Drug Indicators Project at Birkbeck College, London, I worked on a Department of Health and Social Security (DHSS) funded project, examining illicit drug users' perceptions and experiences of a number of statutory and non-statutory services in the central and north London area. By the summer of 1986, the full implications of AIDS for injecting drug users became apparent and we started to question users about their injecting and sharing of equipment, as well as the extent to which concern about AIDS had altered their behaviour. Unless stated otherwise, all the data reported here derive from this research. Whilst not ignoring sexual practices and the cleaning of injecting equipment, the main concern of this chapter is to look at the injecting and needle and syringe sharing patterns amongst injecting drug users, to investigate their responses to the issue of HIV infection and AIDS, and to suggest some strategies that will promote risk reduction. Within these parameters, those who share unsterile injecting equipment are at greatest risk of HIV infection. Drug users who still inject, but who have ceased sharing equipment, can be considered to have substantially reduced their risk behaviour. Those who have never injected cannot have shared, and are only at risk through sexual contact.

Injecting and Sharing Amongst Regular Drug Users

Injecting is a prerequisite for sharing and concomitant high risk behaviour amongst drug users. In the near future, we will have some data on the extent to which injection is employed as a route of administration amongst illicit drug users notified to the Home Office. Since September 1987, and as a direct result of concern about HIV infection and AIDS, all such notifications should contain information on whether or not the drugs concerned were injected. Additionally, a number of research projects are examining the question of injecting drug use and AIDS, and reports from these will in time fill an important gap in our knowledge. Of particular interest will be the findings from the evaluation of the pilot needle and syringe-exchange schemes being conducted by the Monitoring Research Group at

Goldsmiths' College, University of London, and described in Stimson's chapter elsewhere in this book. For the moment, however, no overall picture is available. However, local studies, often with an ethnographic emphasis have pointed to the significance of cultural, social and regional factors in determining patterns in the routes of administration of various drugs and subsequent sharing behaviours. Before examining the effect of AIDS upon injecting and sharing behaviours, it is therefore important to investigate the factors that influence drug users in the choice of their preferred route of administration and consequent sharing of injecting equipment. In the British context, these two related issues can be addressed under the headings of 'pragmatism', 'socialization', and 'circumstance'.

Pragmatism

It is common for individuals to inject illicit drugs on the basis of economic rationale. In Britain, over the last eight years, much of the increase in heroin use has been through people smoking or snorting the drug (Hartnoll, 1986). However, once dependence has been established, and individual habits increase, users often turn to injecting. As one heroin user we have interviewed put it, in simple economic terms: 'To stop me being sick I had to smoke a gram and a half. Now that I'm banging it up, I only need a gram. What would you do?'

Even when smoking is the preferred route of administration, there are times when the substance available is not suitable. Such was the case recently in London regarding heroin. A number of users reported that they had reverted to injecting because the heroin on the market disappeared literally in a puff of smoke. Alternatively, there are times when the opposite is the case. One study in the North of England observed that the arrival of cheap 'brown' heroin from Iran and Pakistan, containing many impurities, led to an increase in smoking, and even a switch from injecting. This resulted partly from the fact that the 'brown' heroin had been especially prepared for smoking, but also because the preparation required to purify it deterred a number of injectors (Pearson, 1987).

Along with pragmatic reasons determining the route of administration, the relative availability of sterile injecting equipment is another factor that influences the likelihood of sharing. Clearly, the introduction of a limited number of needle-exchange schemes will have minimized this problem for a number of drug users. However, these schemes are not accessible to all, and many of the problems associated with obtaining sterile needles still pertain. Until recently in England and Wales, few pharmacists were prepared to sell needles and syringes to drug users. In London, a small number of chemists, spread throughout the capital, were the main suppliers. In Scotland, where a different legal system prevails, legislation inhibited the provision and sale of clean equipment. The 1982 outbreak of hepatitis B in an area of Edinburgh, reported by Robertson *et al.* (1986), was attributed to an increase in the sharing of needles and syringes. This resulted from an acute shortage after the local legal supplier closed, followed by an unofficial prohibition by pharmacists. Of the total sample of 164 studied in this investigation, it was found that 83 per cent had shared or were sharing. On retesting the stored blood samples for HIV antibodies it was found that 51 per cent of the same individuals were seropositive. One response to the situation found in Edinburgh has been the setting up of an alternative counselling and screening clinic for testing injecting drug users for HIV antibodies. In its first year of operation, 441 people were counselled, 60 per cent of whom were injecting drug users or their sexual contacts. Interestingly, and consistent with earlier findings, the HIV seropositivity rate amongst drug users was 52 per cent (Brettle *et al.*, 1987). The connection between needle availability, equipment sharing and HIV infection, has also been made in the American context. In areas where there is a tight control on the supply of syringes, such as in New York City and New Jersey, more than 50 per cent of injecting drug users are estimated to be HIV positive. This compares with estimates of less than 10 per cent in areas such as Chicago and Detroit, where no laws restrict the supply of syringes (*Pharmaceutical Journal*, 1987).

The effects of these kinds of restrictions on supply, and the strategies employed by drug users to obtain injecting equipment, were noted in Haw's (1985) two-year study of Glasgow. Syringes and needles were stolen from hospital dustbins and from doctors' surgeries; or else were bought 'on the street'. Alarmingly, it was found that the practice of sharing equipment was most common amongst recent users, thereby increasing the potential for the rapid spread of infection.

Additionally, the real, or perceived risk to the drug user of obtaining clean equipment is an important pragmatic factor that may lead to sharing. In the past, it has been common for the police to monitor the comings and goings of drug users at chemists known to provide syringes and needles. A high incidence of police intervention and arrests created a very real problem for injecting drug users who might otherwise have utilized these services. Tom is HIV positive, and has a series of convictions for dealing. He always bought his needles and syringes from a well-known chemist in London's West End:

> . . . I'd stopped sharing but still fixed, and I was making a real effort to use clean works. I knew that the police were watching the place, but there was nowhere else to go. Anyway, I'm coming out with my works and I'm stopped by this copper. Next thing I know, I'm in a room they've got round the corner being strip-searched and charged with possession with intent to supply.

Assurances have been made that the police will give the new needle and syringe-exchange schemes a wide berth. The need for the police to allow such schemes to operate relatively unhindered is paramount, as exemplified by the experience of Liverpool (see the chapter by Hart in this book). Such forward thinking should be applauded, and clearly, it is essential that any innovations, be they from government departments or elsewhere, are not frustrated by the vagaries of local policing. Injecting drug users, often suspicious and wary of any new official service, are likely to be deterred from any site they believe to be monitored by the police. Consequently, by not utilizing services that provide sterile injecting equipment, they may become more vulnerable to sharing and possible exposure to infection.

Socialization

Regional and cultural variations have been highlighted as important factors influencing the preferred route of administration of illicit drugs, and the resultant potential for sharing. Robertson *et al.* (1986), Kohn (1985) and Haw (1985) point to the almost exclusive tradition of injecting drug use in Scotland's principal cities of Edinburgh and Glasgow. A couple of hundred miles south-west in Liverpool, Parry (1987) notes that the majority of heroin users smoke, or 'chase the dragon', rather than inject. This, he comments, is in spite of the fact that many may have experimented with injecting. Similarly, in their study of the Wirral, Parker *et al.* (1987) note that the most common route of administration of heroin there was by smoking. Of their sample of 652, 79 per cent smoked the drug, 4 per cent employed injection as the sole route of administration and 11.8 per cent combined injecting with other methods of use. Still in the north of England, Pearson (1987) points to the significance of the traditional route of administering amphetamines in determining injecting patterns of other drugs, especially heroin. Where the injecting of amphetamines and barbiturates was common practice prior to the arrival of cheap heroin in the early 1980s, then it was likely that the newly-available drug itself would be injected. Such was seen to be the case in areas such as Carlisle, where injection was already the dominant feature among poly-drug users of the 1970s. In this context, it is interesting to note renewed concern about the injection of amphetamines users within the context of HIV infection and AIDS. A recent Home Office conference, attended by customs officers, senior police officers and health experts, noted the high rates of injecting amongst these drug users, and the potential for the further spread of infection (*The Independent*, 1987).

In north and central London, our own fieldwork suggests that injecting is still the predominant mode of administration amongst heavy opiate and poly-drug users. Smoking and snorting heroin has been commonly observed amongst casual and less heavy users, as well as amongst recent adolescent users. Amphetamines are both snorted and injected; and cocaine, when not combined with heroin as a 'speedball', is predominantly snorted.

Another aspect of socialization that bears upon injecting and sharing patterns is that of cultural diversity. Although Britain is a multi-ethnic society, very little research has been conducted on drug use amongst minority ethnic groups. This results in part from problems of access, but is also due to the fact that most drug research in Britain has relied on samples obtained from the helping-services, a context in which minority ethnic group members are severely under-represented. However, such information as exists points to the importance of this issue. Our own interviews with a number of black heroin users in London support Pearson (1987) in his contention that although cannabis is commonly used as a social drug within the Afro-Caribbean community, there appears to be a cultural opposition to heroin. Moreover, our interviews suggest there may be cultural barriers to injecting among this group at least. Discussions with a small number of black heroin users indicate that sections of the Afro-Caribbean community and culture may see heroin, and especially the injecting of heroin, as a problem specific to the white population. Black heroin users who inject the drug report being ostracized from their peers, as they are deemed to be turning their backs on their cultural heritage. As Derrick put it 'If you smoke herb you're fine. If you snort coke that's cool. If you mess with smack, you're bad. If you shoot the junk up, you're a white man.' Interestingly, our fieldwork in London's West End indicates high levels of injection amongst the Italian population of drug users, but we have as yet little clear information regarding cultural opinion on this matter. In general, information on the injecting and sharing patterns amongst Britain's ethnic minorities is extremely sparse. Plainly, what is required is in-depth research amongst the various groups to identify the extent of injecting and sharing behaviour, so that appropriate responses can be devised.

Circumstance

Circumstance and situational context play important roles in the injecting and sharing process. Ironically, it is through initiation into injecting that many have their first experience of sharing. Unlike other routes of administering illicit drugs (smoking, inhaling, snorting), injecting not only requires specific technology and equipment, but also necessitates a level of expertise. Early results from research by Hart *et al.* (1987) suggest that 73 per cent of their sample shared needles and syringes on the first occasion of injecting; and Robertson *et al.* (1986) have pointed to the near monopoly that dealers had on injecting equipment in their sample. Confirming this, many drug users interviewed in London report that their first successful injection experience was assisted by another person, most commonly a partner or close friend. In such circumstances the likelihood of sharing is high. Naturally, there is often an expressed feeling of confidence and trust in partners and close friends. Comments like: 'I'd known her for years and it just seemed right to ask her to help me to fix that first time', or 'I have sex with him, so what's the difference if I share works with him?' are common.

Another significant circumstantial factor influencing the potential for sharing is the 'hit or no hit' syndrome. Time and again, drug users being interviewed refer to 'desperation' as a circumstance in which they would be tempted to share. In this context 'desperation' refers to an immediate desire for drugs due to craving or withdrawal. Clean equipment is not readily available, and the individual is vulnerable to sharing. As Jack put it:

> . . . You ask me how has AIDS influenced my sharing? I'll tell you I won't share with anyone. But I know in the back of my mind that if I'm sick and someone offers me gear, and I ain't got a works, then I'll take my chance. AIDS scares me to death, but if it's a hit or no hit, then I'll take the hit . . .

Fieldwork interviews have also pointed to a significant number of injecting drug users who, though not prepared to use other people's injecting equipment, will allow others to use theirs. As one drug user put it:

> . . . There's no way I'm ever going to use another junkie's works. Hep. was bad enough, but AIDS is out of the question. If I've finished with my works and someone asks to use it then that's their business. If they're stupid enough to take the chance then it's none of my concern . . .

This observation is borne out by the findings of Ghodse *et al.* (1987). In their sample of 212 injecting drug users, sixty-four allowed others to use their syringes, and only nineteen reported using other people's.

Along with circumstantial factors, the situational context in which drug use takes place will influence patterns of sharing. From interviews conducted with drug users in prison, it is clear that both drugs and injecting equipment are smuggled in. From prisoners' accounts, it is the latter that is in shortest supply, making the sharing of needles and syringes inevitable, even amongst some of those adamantly against this practice.

Among London's itinerant and often homeless West End drug-using population, the locations for injecting are still the toilets in fast food shops, poolrooms, and other such places where drug users congregate, and where the sharing of available equipment has been commonly observed. There is an added danger here, in that such situations and locations are hardly conducive to the cleansing of equipment between use. At best, needles and syringes are rinsed out, at worst there is not even a tap available to facilitate this. Often individuals believe that what they are doing is sufficient to safeguard them against infection, particularly if they simply pour boiling water over used needles and syringes. In this particular context, it can be argued that 'a little knowledge' can be extremely dangerous.

Similarly, and consistent with Brambill and Maslansky's (1986) observations regarding the lack of opportunity and motivation to thoroughly clean injecting equipment in 'shooting galleries' in New York, was the situation that prevailed in Robertson *et al.*'s (1986)

Edinburgh study. At times equipment was rinsed in tap water, but no serious efforts were made at sterilization. A further risk of infection resulted from the routine practice of 'washout' between injections, whereby blood is drawn back into the syringe after injection, so as to flush out any remaining heroin.

Drug Injection, Risk Behaviour and Concern about AIDS

Drug users change their behaviour for a whole variety of reasons. Without doubt, concern about HIV infection and AIDS is, and will be, a very significant factor influencing this. But as Strang *et al.* (1987) found in their follow-up study of fifty-five drug users in Manchester turned away from treatment, in certain circumstances individuals are capable of moderating their behaviour. Whilst this particular study did not straddle the time period when the risk of HIV infection was becoming more widely recognized, the authors reported that 42 per cent had reduced the frequency of injecting, and that 20 per cent had abstained altogether. Further optimism regarding drug users' potential for behavioural change stems from recent research from the USA. A 1984 study in New York City, at a time when there was no special AIDS education or prevention campaign, found that over 90 per cent of those interviewed knew that the agent responsible for AIDS could be transmitted through the sharing of needles, and 59 per cent reported that they had changed their behaviour to reduce the likelihood of being exposed to infection. In New Jersey, since the latter half of 1985, half of all injecting drug users entering treatment said that AIDS was a prime motivation for their seeking help. Moreover, recent ethnographic work amongst injecting drug users in San Francisco not receiving treatment, found that a 'substantial minority' had decreased their levels of sharing as a direct result of concern over AIDS (Des Jarlais and Friedman, 1987).

Findings like these are echoed by research carried out in London by the Drug Indicators Project. Full details, including the research methodology involved, can be found elsewhere (Power *et al.*, 1988), but findings arising from a preliminary analysis of injecting drug users' behavioural responses to HIV infection will be reported on here. In connection with this work, data from 127 regular illicit drug users have been analyzed. Within this sample, two distinct groups can be distinguished according to their contact, or lack of contact, with services. The first of these, the 'agency group' consisted of those individuals who had been contacted through a number of statutory and non-statutory services located in central and north London. It comprised seventy people (forty-five men and twenty-five women). A second 'non-agency group' of fifty-seven individuals (thirty-three men and twenty-five women) was contacted through 'snowballing', and comprised drug users who had not been in touch with services in the preceding year (if at all), and whose agency contact was minimal. In-depth interviews were carried out with members of both groups. These interviews investigated injecting behaviours, and questions were asked about changes in injecting practices and needle and syringe sharing patterns. Respondents were asked who, if anyone, they shared with, how regularly this occurred, and the degree to which concern about AIDS had been influential in any changes. Also information on testing for HIV antibody status was gathered.

Amongst those who had ever injected, it was found that 54 per cent had substantially reduced their risk behaviour, in that they either no longer injected, or else no longer shared needles or syringes. A further 32 per cent had to some extent reduced their risk behaviour, and only 14 per cent stated that they had been unaffected by concern about AIDS. Those who were in contact with agencies were more likely to have substantially reduced their risk behaviour than those not in contact with agencies. Similarly, and although the numbers were small, the results tended to suggest that those who had been tested for HIV were more likely to be amongst those who had substantially reduced their risks than those who had not been tested.

Conclusions

The above findings lead to a number of conclusions. First, regional and cultural variations in both injecting and sharing habits must be taken into account when devising preventative or risk reduction strategies. Different approaches are needed in an area, or amongst groups, where smoking or snorting illicit drugs is the common practice, as opposed to another context where injecting and sharing is firmly established. It is essential that reliable knowledge is obtained about the behaviours and patterns amongst specific groups of drug users, so that appropriate responses are employed. This is especially the case amongst members of minority ethnic groups in Britain, where little is known about drug use and patterns of injecting. Individuals who would be freely accepted by these groups, could be employed to work in both a research and AIDS-health outreach capacity. None of this is to deny that, with regard to AIDS and patterns of injecting, there are central messages to convey, and habits common to many to alter. Rather, it is to highlight the need for sensitivity to regional and cultural variation.

Second, it should be recognized that some people will not only continue to abuse illicit drugs, but will also continue to inject and share equipment. Research at St. Mary's Hospital, London, amongst 114 drug users receiving treatment, has suggested that the main factor influencing sharing is the availability of needles and syringes. Of those injectors who were HIV antibody positive, 64 per cent gave this answer, and amongst the HIV antibody negative sample, 72 per cent mentioned this as their prime reason for sharing (Mulleady, 1987). Therefore, clean needles and syringes must be made freely available so as to break the connection between scarcity of injecting equipment, needle sharing and infection. The needle-exchange schemes should prove to be a step in the right direction. Other schemes, such as those operating in Bradford, where twenty-three pharmacists cooperated in the provision of clean needles, condoms, advice and information to drug users, should also be encouraged (Marfell *et al.*, 1987). To complement initiatives like these, appropriate information regarding safe sex practices and the cleaning of injecting equipment should be made available nationally to injecting drug users. Regarding this latter point, the practical problems facing drug users who endeavour to sterilize needles and syringes, and conflicting advice about the most effective methods, mean that at present this strategy for risk reduction has serious drawbacks. It should not, therefore, be seen as a panacea in itself, but as part of a broader strategy of health education.

It must be acknowledged, however, that a substantial proportion of injectors do not use established drug services, neither do they use existing needle-exchange schemes. Preliminary results from our own research have shown that those in touch with services are more likely to have reduced their risk behaviour. This may either be because their contact with professionals has encouraged behavioural change, or it may result from the fact that a greater concern about AIDS leads to agency contact. While these are questions for further investigation, the fact that the 'non-agency group' forms a higher proportion of those in the high risk category, means that there is a clear need for aggressive outreach work. Urgent contact with drug injectors at high risk of sharing and HIV infection needs to be made in the community, and sterile injecting equipment and appropriate health education material needs to be provided on a regular basis. Only when such steps are taken, can we be said to be making progress towards a truly comprehensive programme of harm minimization and risk reduction.

Acknowledgement

The first section of this chapter is a revised and updated version of a paper presented at a NIDA Technical Meeting held in Washington DC, USA, May 1987.

References

BRAMBILL, B. and MASLANSKY, R. (1986) 'AIDS and the intravenous drug abuser', *Journal of Substance Abuse Treatment*, 3, 3, p 155.
BRETTLE, R., BISSET, K. and BURNS, S. *et al.* (1987) 'Human immunodeficiency virus and drug misuse: The Edinburgh experience', *British Medical Journal*, 295, pp 421–4.
DES JARLAIS, D. and FRIEDMAN, S. (1987) 'Target groups for preventing AIDS among intravenous drug users', *Journal of Applied Social Psychology*, 17, 3, pp 251–68.
GHODSE, A., TREGENGA, G. and LI, M. (1987) 'Effect of fear of AIDS on sharing of injecting equipment among drug abusers', *British Medical Journal*, 295, pp 698–9.
HART, G., PETHERICK, A. and SONNEX, C. (1987) personal communication, Middlesex Hospital Medical School, University of London.
HARTNOLL, R. L. (1986) 'Recent trends in drug use in Britain', *Druglink*, 1, 2, pp 10–11.
HAW, S. (1985) *Drug problems in Greater Glasgow*, London, Standing Conference on Drug Abuse.
KOHN, M. (1986) 'The virus in Edinburgh', *New Society*, 2 May, pp 11–13.
MARFELL, K., MITCHELL-CHRISTIE, A., JOHNSON, A. and HINDS, G. (1987) 'Needle exchange and HIV infection', *Lancet*, pp 100–1.
MULLEADY, G. (1987) unpublished paper, London, St. Mary's Hospital.
PARKER, H., NEWCOMBE, R. and BATX, K. (1987) 'The new heroin users: Prevalence and characteristics in Wirral, Merseyside', *British Journal of Addiction*, 82, 20, pp 147–57.
PARRY, A. (1987) 'Needle swop in Mersey', *Druglink*, 2, 1, p 7.
PEARSON, G. (1987) *The New Heroin Users*, Oxford, Basil Blackwell.
Pharmaceutical Journal (1987) 18 July, p 66.
POWER, R., HARTNOLL, R. and DAVIAUD, E. (1988) 'Drug injecting, AIDS and risk reduction: Potential for change and intervention strategies', *British Journal of Addiction*, 83, pp 649–54.
ROBERTSON, J. R., BUCKNALL, A. B. V. and WELSBY, P. D. *et al.* (1986)

'Epidemic of AIDS, related virus (HTLV-III/LAV) infection among intravenous drug abusers', *British Medical Journal*, 292, pp 527–9.
STRANG, J., HEATHCOTE, S. and WATSON, P. (1987) 'Habit moderation in injecting drug addicts', *Health Trends*, 19, 3, pp 16–8.
The Independent (1987) 14 March, p 2.

11
Syringe-Exchange Schemes in England and Scotland: Evaluating a New Service for Drug Users

Gerry V. Stimson, Lindsey Alldritt, Kate Dolan and Martin Donoghue

Early in 1987, the UK government launched a number of schemes to attempt to reduce the spread of HIV infection amongst injecting drug users. These schemes make syringes and needles available to users, together with advice on drug use and safer sex. They are commonly known as syringe or needle-exchange schemes. The introduction of this new policy marked a change of direction with respect to the desirability or otherwise of distributing injecting equipment to drug users. Only a year before there had been little official support for making syringes and needles freely available (Short, 1986), which made the speed with which syringe exchanges were introduced all the more surprising. The schemes themselves were launched in April 1987, a mere four months after a government decision had been made. This chapter will examine the background to the introduction of these schemes and the manner in which they were set up. It will also present preliminary findings from an evaluation of their work being carried out by the Monitoring Research Group at Goldsmiths' College, London.

The Background

While reliable statistics are hard to come by, it is currently estimated about 60,000 people inject drugs in Britain today. As is discussed elsewhere in this book (see the chapters by Hart, Power and Mulleady), many injecting drug users may be at a high risk of HIV infection primarily because of the sharing of equipment. There are high levels of sharing in some parts of Britain (Advisory Council on the Misuse of Drugs, 1988; Des Jarlais and Friedman, 1985), and it is now well established that the high level of HIV infection amongst injecting drug users in cities such as Edinburgh is directly attributable to this particular practice. Moreover, data from Edinburgh point to the rapidity with which infection can spread amongst those who share needles and syringes. Two years after HIV infection was first recorded amongst the city's injecting drug users, up to half of those tested were HIV antibody positive (Robertson *et al.*, 1986).

There is, however, considerable variation on this pattern nationally and regionally and care should be taken in the interpretation of HIV seropositivity rates amongst injecting drug users due to variable coverage and differences in sampling. Nevertheless, on the basis of present knowledge (which is still scanty), parts of Scotland continue to have higher seropositivity rates than elsewhere in the country. Whereas in England and Wales and Northern Ireland, injecting drug users make up less than 10 per cent of the cumulative reported total of HIV antibody positive persons, in Scotland they constitute the largest single group, comprising 58 per cent of reported cases by September 1987.

In some parts of the country, however, the incidence of HIV infection amongst injecting drug users is still low. In Glasgow, for example, a rate of 4.5 per cent was recorded in 1985 (Follett *et al.*, 1986), and rates of between 0 and 10 per cent have recently been reported in various towns in England (Advisory Council on the Misuse of Drugs, 1988). If these reports provide a reliable estimate of actual rates then, whilst the potential for a serious situation exists, in many areas there is still time for preventive action.

In England, Wales and Northern Ireland, 5 per cent of those reported as HIV antibody positive are women: most of them are injecting drug users. In Scotland, on the other hand, 26 per cent of reported cases of HIV infection are women: again, most of them are injecting drug users. In all parts of Britain, the proportion of men to women amongst HIV antibody positive persons who inject is approximately 2 : 1, whereas most studies of injecting drug use suggest that the proportion of men to women overall is in the region of 3 : 1.

The main mode of HIV transmission amongst injecting drug users is through the sharing of equipment such as needles and syringes; the relative importance of sexual transmission amongst those who inject is currently less well understood. Whilst there is still much to be learned about the behavioural aspects of transmission, it is now clear that apart from the numbers of persons already infected, the availability (or otherwise) of clean injecting equipment is a key factor in determining the extent to which infection is spread. Nevertheless, it is not just availability that matters. In Italy, for example, where clean equipment is readily available, there are still high rates of HIV infection amongst injecting drug users. This suggests that knowledge about the steps that can be taken to avoid infection is also important.

Traditional Patterns of Syringe Availability

In the United Kingdom, syringes are available for retail purchase in pharmacy shops, and pharmacists use their discretion regarding syringe sales. In 1982, in an attempt to help reduce the increase in the number of drug users, pharmacists were recommended by their professional society to restrict sales to *bona fide* patients for therapeutic purposes only. In effect, this was a recommendation not to sell to drug users, although it should be noted that not all pharmacists followed this advice. In 1986, in view of evidence linking HIV infection and AIDS to the sharing of equipment, this recommendation was withdrawn (*Pharmaceutical Journal*, 1986). Since then, pharmacists have been encouraged to reconsider their role *vis-à-vis* injecting drug use, and to give careful consideration to sales of syringes (National Pharmaceutical Association, 1986). In practice however, some retail pharmacists remain unwilling to sell syringes to drug users, mostly because they fear that the presence of injecting drug users on their premises may deter other customers.

In Scotland, the legal position regarding syringe sales by pharmacists is less clear because of the common law offence of reckless conduct. Several successful prosecutions have been brought against shopkeepers on the grounds that they have recklessly supplied children with solvents in the knowledge that they intend to inhale them. No charges have so far been brought against any pharmacist in Scotland for selling syringes to drug misusers. However there have been reports that police in some parts of Scotland had been active in dissuading pharmacists from this kind of activity.

Changes in Policy

Reports of high levels of HIV infection among Scottish injecting drug users (Peutherer *et al.*, 1985; Robertson *et al.*, 1986) were significant in influencing the decision by the Scottish Home and Health Department (SHHD) in 1986 to establish the McClelland Committee. The McClelland Report, published in September of that year, considered that police activity in Edinburgh discouraging the sale of syringes and needles was possibly an important factor influencing the spread of HIV in the city. The Committee felt that 'the resultant non-availability of sterile equipment in the city, appears to have contributed to extensive sharing of equipment'. Additionally, it was suggested that a low level of investment in treatment services may have led many drug users to avoid seeking professional help. The report concluded (amongst other things) that steps should be taken to provide sterile injecting equipment and counselling to those who were unwilling or unable to stop injecting.

Issues raised in the McClelland Report and concern about the spread of HIV were subsequently taken up by officials in both the SHHD and the Department of Health and Social Security (DHSS). In December 1986 the Secretary of State for Social Services announced first the provision of £1m in 1987/88 to enable drug agencies to enhance their counselling services on AIDS and drug misuse, and second the establishment of a number of special needle-exchange and counselling schemes (DHSS, 1986). The Minister of State for Scotland announced at the same time that special schemes in Scotland would also be established, and £300,000 would be made available to enable drug agencies to enhance their counselling services on AIDS and drug misuse.

This is not the place to go into detail about recent developments in British drugs policy except to note that concurrent with an increased centralism in policy making in general, there have been similar moves in the drugs field. Here, traditional forms of policy making based on advice from professional workers have to some extent been displaced in favour of central government initiatives (Stimson, 1987). Government policies in the drugs field have been implemented for the most part by advisory statements, and by monetary incentives in the form of short term 'pump priming' for favoured projects, after which responsibility for funding is shifted to other agencies. This strategy has enabled a quick response to some drug problems, of which the response to HIV and drug use is a good example.

The first public announcements about the proposed injection-equipment schemes came in December 1986. The DHSS subsequently invited existing drug agencies to establish schemes on a pilot one-year basis, with offers of some financial support for the first year of their operation. This invitation went to agencies in the health service such as drug dependency clinics, as well as other drug agencies outside the National Health Service (NHS) such as information and advice agencies. In Scotland, the SHHD asked health boards to set up the schemes.

There was not unanimous support for the schemes. Following close on the DHSS's 1986 anti-heroin campaign, and in the context of broader government strategies to tackle drug misuse, critics might have claimed some inconsistency in the provision of a service that enabled the continued use of illicit drugs. Concern was also expressed that increasing the availability of syringes might lead to an increase in the number of injectors, so that even if the rates of HIV infection amongst injecting drug users did not increase, there would still be absolute increases in the number infected. The schemes were therefore launched on a pilot basis with the guarantee that their operation would be evaluated. In setting up the schemes, the DHSS stipulated that the following requirements should be met. Participating agencies should:

(a) issue injecting equipment on an exchange basis to drug misusers already injecting and unable or unwilling to stop;
(b) provide assessment of, and counselling for, clients' drug problems;
(c) provide advice on safe sex, and offer counselling in connection with HIV antibody testing;
(d) collect information on clients and collaborate with a monitoring/evaluation project.

The Exchange Schemes

In Britain, there have been officially sanctioned forms of syringe distribution since the late 1960s, when injecting equipment was given to drug users receiving prescribed injectable drugs. The idea that there should be exchange schemes however resurfaced in October 1986 during a conference in Sweden organized by the World Health Organization (WHO). Amidst growing awareness of HIV and of the success of the Amsterdam syringe-distribution schemes (whose operation in fact predates more recent concern about AIDS), it was felt that initiatives of this kind could have an important role to play in stopping the spread of HIV amongst injecting drug users (WHO, 1987). As a result, by the time the government announced the schemes, a few (such as those in Liverpool and Sheffield) were already in operation, and these were among those drawn into the 'official' response. The formal start of the schemes was however in April 1987.

Initially fifteen agencies in England and Scotland were recruited to run pilot injecting equipment exchange schemes (there are also some other schemes outside the 'official' ones) and the rest of this chapter concentrates on their experience during their first few months of operation up to September 1987.

Syringe-exchange schemes vary considerably in their operation. Some are linked to out-patient drug dependency clinics. Others can be found outside the NHS in drug advice and information agencies. Most are office based, but one involves local pharmacists in distribution, after clients have first been screened by the drug agency. One started operation in the Accident and Emergency department of a large city hospital. Most are open office hours, but not all are open every day.

Accommodation is often minimal — it may be a corner of a room that has other uses, or a small room set aside for the purpose. For example, the Liverpool scheme was run during its first year from a converted toilet on the ground floor of a drug information agency. The Edinburgh scheme runs from an out-patient clinic in Leith Hospital, and at other times in the week the accommodation is used for a child health clinic. In Sheffield, where the scheme is based in pharmacies, the exchange operates from the pharmacist's counter.

Operating costs are relatively small. First there is the cost of injecting equipment itself. This will include the syringes, which retail at about 14p each, and condoms. Then there is staff time, which ranges from a part-time post to two posts, depending on the scale of the scheme. Staff are community psychiatric nurses, ordinary nurses or social workers, and in Scotland include doctors.

The basic system is that new clients must show evidence of injecting drug use and an unwillingness or inability to stop injecting. Once drug users have been accepted into the scheme, they are given injecting equipment. This is usually available in a choice of barrel and needle sizes. Some schemes also provide sterile water, and material for cleaning the skin before injection. On subsequent visits, clients return their used injecting equipment. This is counted and placed in a safe container for later destruction, and new equipment is issued, usually on a one-to-one basis. A record is taken of the transaction. The number of needles and syringes issued at any one time varies, but is in the region of five to ten. In Scotland, a maximum of three syringes is issued on any one occasion. There will also be counselling for clients on drug use and safer sex, but not on every visit. Condoms are provided by some schemes. In all but one agency, the service and equipment are free to the client.

Legal Issues

Some of the legal issues relating to the schemes have already been touched on earlier in the discussion of syringe availability. One problem for staff and clients is that the possession of used syringes with drug traces can be used by the police in prosecutions for the illegal possession of drugs. It was originally thought that this problem might deter clients from returning used syringes and in consequence, consultations have taken place between the government and Chief Constables, and drugs agencies and the local police. In general though, the police have agreed to cooperate with the schemes subject to their obligation to uphold the law. The government has also attempted to influence prosecution policies. The Attorney General recently announced that 'When reaching decisions in cases relating to misuse of drugs, the Crown prosecution service, where relevant, will have proper regard to public interest considerations arising out of the measures brought in to halt the spread of the AIDS virus' (Hansard, 1987). In Liverpool, police finding someone in possession of a used syringe will confiscate the syringe and give the user a receipt which can be used to obtain fresh equipment from the exchange scheme.

As we have seen, in Scotland it was originally feared that agency staff might be liable to prosecution under the common law. The Lord Advocate has, however, indicated that doctors and staff participating in the schemes will be immune from prosecution if they follow the procedures approved for the schemes.

Progress with the Schemes

From their inception, it was intended that their operation should be monitored and evaluated. It would seem appropriate therefore to report on preliminary findings from research carried out by the Monitoring Research Group at Goldsmiths' College, London which was charged with this responsibility.

Some of the schemes have been very successful in attracting clients. Between them, the fifteen schemes have attracted over 1500 clients in the period up until September 1987. They differ, however, in their ability to attract clients. One of the longer established schemes, for example, has seen nearly 700 different clients in its first year of operation, and even some of those more recently opened are drawing in large numbers of clients. One of these in London has been seeing up to fifty people in a day. Others have not attracted such large numbers, however, and there are several which have had less than ten clients.

The schemes draw in a wide range of different types of clients. What is most significant in this respect is that they attract people who are not in touch with other drug services. The majority have had either no prior contact with drug services, or are not in current contact with them. Clients are predominantly male (indeed more so than in most other drug-using groups), mainly using heroin — though with a sizeable number using amphetamine — and have on average several years from the time they first injected drugs to their first attendance at the scheme.

On the whole, the schemes have shown that they are able to get syringes to drug injectors, and to get them returned. Our best estimate is that approximately 45,000 syringes have been distributed since the start of the schemes. Return rates vary between 30 to 100 per cent of those issued.

Two Schemes Examined

Two schemes have been in operation since before the 'official' start of the programme in April 1987. The activities of these will be used to indicate some of the different ways in which exchange schemes can operate.

Liverpool has high levels of heroin use and drug-related crime (Parker *et al*, 1987), and its syringe-exchange scheme started in October 1986, launched by a local drug training and information service which does not normally involve itself directly in client work (Parry, 1987). The service is operated in a converted bathroom on the ground floor near the main entrance to the building and is open office hours. Clients are seen first by the receptionist, who then refers them to one of the available syringe-exchange workers. New clients are asked to produce evidence of injection sites.

At first, many of the clients of this scheme were patients receiving treatment at the drug dependency clinic next door. Since then, news of the exchange service offered by the drug training and information service has spread by word of mouth and media advertising. Leaflets are distributed in the city on AIDS and injecting drugs, and the scheme also provides individual counselling on safer drug use and injection practices and safer sex. Overall, the scheme has developed into a 'consumer advice' service for drug users with an operating philosophy of harm reduction.

Between December 1986 and August 1987, 617 clients had been to the scheme, but just over half of these (51 per cent) had visited the scheme once only. There is an average of fifteen exchanges per day. An average of ten syringe barrels is issued, with extra needles, and both are offered in a choice of three sizes. Clients are also given swabs, condoms and spermicides. Over this period, nearly 28,000 syringes were distributed. Returning clients show staff their used syringes and then place them in a safe container. Clients wanting HIV testing are referred to the local Genito-Urinary Medicine Clinic (Newcombe *et al.*, 1987).

Sheffield's scheme on the other hand involves pharmacists. There are estimated to be about 1500 injecting drug users in South Yorkshire, and in Sheffield the main drug injected is heroin. The idea for a syringe-exchange scheme was first raised by local pharmacists who asked the local drugs agency for advice after being asked for syringes by drug injectors. The scheme that was eventually established in June 1986 involved six local pharmacists who agreed to sell syringes on an exchange basis. Anyone who approaches a pharmacist for syringes is referred first by the pharmacists to one of the two local drug advice projects. There, the person's drug use is assessed, and if it is agreed that the person should be supplied with syringes, they are referred back to the pharmacist with a letter of authorization.

In fact, much of the work is now concentrated in two pharmacies, one of which is part of a large national chain. Approximately eighty clients have been enrolled, but the number of regular attenders is about twenty per week at each pharmacy. The pharmacist reports little difficulty in the arrangement. There have been minimal comments from other customers, but some shoplifting. It is notable that in this 'commercial' scheme there is less advice-seeking from clients, and less counselling given. The clients see it primarily as a shopkeeping transaction.

A Preliminary Assessment of the Schemes

Many of the schemes have only been running for a short time and are still establishing reputations and working practices. It is too soon therefore to draw firm conclusions about their value. However, a number of issues can be identified that are worthy of discussion and further investigation.

First, whilst some schemes attract large numbers of clients, others have failed to do so. There are a number of reasons for this, not all of which apply to every scheme. One of the rural schemes, for example, has a scattered drug-using population with sporadic injecting related to fluctuations in drug supplies. In some cities, pharmacists may traditionally have been willing suppliers of syringes and needles. Some schemes may not have received enough publicity or a high enough profile on the local grapevine. Others may have problems of accessibility due to their geographical and institutional location, the most accessible are placed in high drug use areas with access being gained from the street.

Second, schemes vary in the quality of the relationships they establish with clients. This can best be described by the term used by some agencies — 'user friendliness'. The schemes that are most successful in attracting clients appear to be those where staff are non-judgmental and lack the coerciveness that characterizes many client–professional encounters.

Third, some staff have begun to rethink the character of their work with drug users. All schemes operate with a risk reduction philosophy, that is, they aim to counsel drug users to change their injecting and sexual behaviour in order to reduce the risk of HIV infection. But at a few of them the staff have developed a broader harm-minimization approach that involves tackling other problems that clients might face from injecting themselves or from their drug use. For example longer-term drug injectors with damaged veins may need advice on new sites. Syringe-exchange workers thus have to face the issue of whether to teach people how to inject in a safer way. Not everyone is able to work in this way. Some staff have personal doubts about the desirability of syringe-exchange, or pursuing harm-minimization to the extent of teaching drug users how to inject. Their doubts must be placed in the context of the way in which British drug treatment policy has developed in the last few years, which has been oriented to contract therapy and abstinence. It is hard for some drug workers to adopt the very different style of work required by harm-minimization.

Fourth, most schemes run syringe-exchange in a different location to other services. Syringe-exchange does not fit easily with other services on the same site (although there are exceptions), since it can create conflicts between clients, and conflicts for staff who may have to operate different approaches for different groups of clients. But although it seems best that schemes should stand alone, syringe-exchange schemes are not substitutes for other services, and need to be able to refer people to more specialist workers as appropriate. Integrated syringe-exchange schemes can therefore be seen as a 'low-threshold' contact point for drug users.

Fifth, the schemes are identifying a wide range of problems in clients that are not being dealt with satisfactorily by other agencies. Significant here is the lack of primary health care for many drug injectors, and numerous social welfare and drug related problems. Some syringe-exchange workers find they spend much of their time trying to get such help for clients.

Sixth, the extent, intensity and quality of counselling is extremely variable. It is mainly provided in an *ad hoc* way — when the opportunity arises. Some schemes have developed clear counselling strategies, others have yet to address this. Most agencies and clients find it harder to discuss sexual practices than to discuss drug use. Indeed, when clients have been interviewed about the behavioural changes they have made 'because of AIDS', twice as many report some change in drug use practice as report changes in sexual practice.

Seventh, the position of syringe-exchange in Scotland to date appears to be particularly problematic. One of the pilot schemes has now closed, and another (in Glasgow) faced a picket by local residents who objected to its location. These problems arise from a combination of factors including administrative and financial uncertainties, the geographical and institutional location of schemes, and the operating philosophy of the staff. Furthermore, legal problems, and consequent limits on the number of syringes distributed on any one occasion, combined with limited opening times, are not conducive to successful operation. Despite these hindrances, the Scottish schemes are seeing more clients than some of those in England.

Eighth, the lack of public opposition to the schemes is noteworthy. Other than in Glasgow, where local residents opposed the originally proposed location for the scheme, and where the new site has also faced a local residents' picket, there has been little organized public opposition. In some environments, this may be due to a lack of public awareness, although this is not the whole picture because some schemes have had considerable local publicity. In one town for example, an advertisement for the schemes went out with the local rate demands. In others there has been considerable local media coverage.

Ninth, the police have cooperated with the operation of many schemes. Some forces have decided against using drug traces in syringes as forensic evidence for possession apart from exceptional cases. This policy may in part be connected with the increasing reluctance of forensic scientists to handle syringes. Many forces have agreed to cooperate with the schemes. At least one force has a policy of confiscating syringes, but for which a receipt is issued and the person given details of the syringe exchange.

Finally, it is important to reflect on the ability of the schemes to reach enough people. Some schemes have, in a short time, reached large numbers of people, many of whom are not reached by other services. Other things being equal, the total capacity of the pilot schemes would be in the range of 2000 to 3500 different clients per annum. This is a good achievement. But with upwards of 60,000 regular drug injectors in this country it will need a major expansion of the schemes to reach sufficient numbers of drug injectors. There will also be those who never approach them, for even the most user friendly schemes may seem intimidating to some clients. Syringe-exchange can then, be only one part of a package of responses that must be developed to stem the spread of HIV in injecting drug users.

Acknowedgements

The research on which this chapter draws is funded by the Department of Health and Social Security. The contribution of co-workers Lindsey Alldritt, Kate Dolan and Martin Donoghoe is acknowledged.

References

Advisory Council on the Misuse of Drugs (1988) *Report: AIDS and Drug Misuse, Part I*, London, Department of Health and Social Security, HMSO.

Des Jarlais, D.C. and Friedman, S.R. (1985) 'Risk reduction for AIDS among intravenous drug users', *Ann. Intern. Med.*, 103, 5, pp 755–9.

DHSS (1986) 'New measures to fight the spread of AIDS', press release 86/418.

FOLLETT, E. A., WALLACE, L. A. and McCRUDEN, E. A. (1986) 'HIV and HBV infection in drug abusers in Glasgow', *Lancet*, 1, p 920.

HANSARD (1987) report in *Druglink*, May/June.

NATIONAL PHARMACEUTICAL ASSOCIATION (1986) 'The dilemma — drug addicts and AIDS', *The Supplement*, p 690.

NEWCOMBE, R., PARRY, A. and CARR, J. (1987) 'Syringe-exchange schemes for drug injectors: Reducing the spread of HIV infection and other harm', *mimeo*.

PARKER, H., NEWCOMBE, R. and BAKX, K. (1987) 'The new heroin users: Prevalence and characteristics in Wirral, Merseyside', *British Journal of Addiction*, 82, pp 147–57.

PARRY, A. (1987) 'Needle swap in Mersey', *Druglink*, January/February, p 7.

PEUTHERER, J. F., EDMOND, E., SIMMONDS, P., DICKSON, J. D. and BATH, G. E. (1985) 'HTLV-III antibody in Edinburgh drug addicts', *Lancet*, p 1129.

Pharmaceutical Journal (1986) 'Council statement: Sale of hypodermic syringes and needles', p 205.

ROBERTSON, J. R., BUCKNALL, A. B. V. and WELSBY, P. D. *et al* (1986) 'Epidemic of AIDS related virus (HTLV-III/LAV) infection among intravenous drug abusers', *British Medical Journal*, 292, p 527.

SHHD (1986) *HIV Infection in Scotland: Report of the Scottish Committee on HIV Infection and Intravenous Drug Misuse*, Edinburgh, SHHD.

SHORT, R. (1986) 'Health summary', *Times Health Supplement*, 9 March.

STIMSON, G. V. (1987) 'British drug policies in the 1980s: A preliminary assessment and suggestions for research', *British Journal of Addiction*, 82, pp 477–88.

WHO (1987) *AIDS Among Drug Abusers*, Copenhagen, WHO Regional Office for Europe.

12
Injecting Drug Use and HIV Infection — Intervention Strategies for Harm Minimization

Geraldine Mulleady, Graham Hart and Peter Aggleton

In this chapter we will review some of the different strategies that can be used to reduce the spread of HIV infection amongst injecting drug users. All of these are based upon the concept of 'harm-minimization'. Harm-minimization has two complementary dimensions: the first, which falls into the category of primary prevention, involves persuading individuals not to start injecting illicit drugs. The second aims to reduce the harm associated with injecting drug use, both for the individual and the community.

In fact, as is suggested by Hart elsewhere in this book, some workers in the drugs field do not see these approaches as complementary at all, perceiving them instead as mutually exclusive. In this chapter, we will draw on the experience gained by one of us (Mulleady) working in the St. Mary's Hospital Drug Dependency Unit, to suggest that, within the context of HIV infection, it may be possible to work with drug users in such a way so as to discourage drug use by not actively supporting it, whilst ensuring that for those who do continue to use illicit drugs, every opportunity is made available to reduce the personal and social consequences of this activity.

The particular kind of intervention that is most appropriate for a given individual will depend on many factors, including the extent to which she or he is at risk of HIV infection. In this context, level of risk can be conceived as a continuum along which an individual's behaviour can be placed, ranging from high risk involving sharing needles and syringes and having unprotected penetrative intercourse, to low risk behaviour such as the single use of new needles and syringes and having safer sex. We will argue that after assessing an individual's knowledge regarding the transmission of HIV and by employing non-threatening and non-judgmental questions regarding level of risk, it is possible to respond with interventions which will introduce or maintain, as appropriate, low risk behaviour.

Behavioural Change

There is only limited and often anecdotal knowledge about the behaviour of injecting drug users prior to the identification of AIDS (Howard and Borges, 1970). Although original research is now taking place into the behaviour of this population (much of this is described elsewhere in this book) the potential threat posed by the spread of HIV infection is such that, when designing prevention programmes, health care professionals must often rely on research findings that are far from conclusive.

Nevertheless, preliminary findings from studies carried out in the United States and Northern Europe suggest that, in the context of AIDS, substantial numbers of injecting drug users have modified at least some of their HIV transmission behaviours. In New York, for example, 54 per cent of injecting drug users in a study undertaken in 1984 reported that they had reduced their high risk injection practices (Des Jarlais *et al.*, 1984), whilst Selwyn *et al.* (1985) identified a 60 per cent reduction in risk behaviour, with most users reporting a reduction in needle sharing.

Although caution must be exercised when undertaking cross-national comparisons of the behaviour of drug users, not least because of variations in local legal sanctions and policing policies, some relatively clear patterns of response to HIV amongst drug users in different cultures can be identified. In San Francisco, for example, 73 per cent of drug users had made at least one change in their drug related behaviour, such as not sharing or sharing equipment less frequently, in order to avoid exposure to HIV (Newmeyer *et al.*, 1988). In Amsterdam, Bunning *et al.* (1987) found that amongst 150 injecting drug users surveyed, needle sharing had fallen from approximately 70 per cent engaged in this activity in the early eighties to 20 per cent in 1987. In a study of injecting drug users attending St. Mary's Drug Dependency Unit in 1987 it was found that of seventy-four clients 65 per cent reported that they had shared syringes previously, but were not now doing so because of AIDS (Mulleady and Sherr, 1988). Unfortunately, by way of contrast, there were few indications of there being any significant reduction in high risk sexual behaviour. This reaffirms the importance of not neglecting the sexual dimension of risk reduction amongst drug users.

What kinds of options are available to health care professionals as service providers, and injecting drug users as consumers to facilitate individual and group risk reduction? In this chapter, we will identify a variety of interventions that can be used either individually or in combination, depending on the individual's particular needs. These include approaches such as Methadone treatment and HIV antibody testing which have the individual as their focus, as well as those that aim to affect drug users as a group. The latter include syringe-exchange schemes and outreach work which, whilst certainly having consequences for individuals, are clearly part of a broader public health strategy to resist the further spread of HIV infection. At first sight, the aims of some of these interventions might appear contradictory, for example, the provision of clean needles to people on Methadone programmes. Nevertheless, if risk reduction is to be our primary goal, interventions must be tailored to the reality of drug users' experience to be successful.

Methadone Treatment

It is worth considering Methadone briefly from an historical perspective. This synthetic opiate (opioid) has been variously considered to be either a universal panacea or an unmitigated evil. Sadly, the majority of arguments for and against its therapeutic value derive from studies carried out in the pre-AIDS era, many of which were plagued by methodological problems (Gossop, 1987). Research of this kind attempted to determine if Methadone was an effective treatment in its own right (often with drug abuse being conceived of as a 'metabolic disease'), or whether it was only useful as an adjunct to other forms of treatment, such as psychotherapy. This is a debate which has re-emerged with respect to the role of Methadone in HIV and drug abuse.

Little reassurance can be found in published research, with its conflicting findings and resultant uncertainties. For example, there is little evidence that dosage levels are crucial to successful outcomes in terms of the period following treatment being drug-free (Goldstein, 1971; Connell, 1975). One study found that maintenance on a low dosage did better than a high dosage (20–70 mgs) in terms of social adaptation measures and reduction in illicit drug use (Schut, File and Wohlmuth, 1973). Moreover, Methadone's ability to retain clients in treatment has also been questioned with Williams and Lee (1975) finding that only 25 per cent of their sample remained in treatment. Hartnoll *et al.* (1980) compared clients receiving oral Methadone with those on intravenous heroin maintenance, and found no difference between the two groups in terms of use of illicit opiates, employment and patterns of health. However, the heroin group did show a better attendance rate (75 per cent of the heroin group compared to 29 per cent of the Methadone group after twelve months).

Methadone treatment is reportedly popular with drug users according to many Drug Dependency Unit workers. In the absence of research in this area, however, it is difficult to determine the extent to which this may be due to the perceived value of Methadone or to the absence of other opiate-based treatments in many clinics. Who would ask for wine in a bar known only to stock beer?

Much of the research into the effectiveness of Methadone treatment was carried out prior to the epidemic of HIV infection. It is therefore clearly inappropriate to uncritically apply findings from this period to the present situation. Preliminary findings from research into the role of Methadone maintenance programmes in reducing transmission related behaviours has in fact indicated that drug users on such regimes may inject less frequently than those who are not (Des Jarlais and Friedman, 1987).

Apart from further funding and an expansion of services, increased access to Methadone treatment programmes could be achieved if time-consuming assessment procedures were streamlined. Such an approach has been adopted at the Northern Road Drug Clinic in Portsmouth. The programme here is designed in three stages. The drug user has quick access to stage one of the programme where they collect their Methadone from the clinic for a set period. At the time of collection, if they wish, the drug user has access to an open-ended discussion group which uses motivational interviewing techniques (Van Bilsen, 1986). There are no further programme constraints. Should the client decide that they want to reduce their Methadone intake or come off the drug entirely, they can proceed to stage 2 where they can pick up Methadone daily from a local chemist and attend the clinic for urine assessment and counselling. There is also a third option which combines more flexible access to Methadone with a reduced frequency of attendance at the clinic. The Portsmouth programme is community-based, with staff making regular home visits — a change of practice brought about as a result of the clinic's response to HIV, and one which has increased the rate of referrals.

Although this style of intervention may not be universally appropriate, certain aspects of it could be adopted by other clinics. It also provides a rare example of a treatment unit being prepared to radically change existing policies and procedures. There is a need for increased coordination of our approach to drug treatment, incorporating sensitivity to local needs. Present systems are often unable to respond effectively to the changing circumstances of the people for whom services are provided.

HIV Antibody Testing

While it has often been suggested that HIV antibody testing can have a significant influence on transmission related behaviour in drug users, only limited evidence is so far available to enable us to evaluate these claims (Casadonte *et al.*, 1986; Cox *et al.*, 1986; Marlink, 1987). In the short term, these studies evidence a dramatic reduction in needle sharing behaviour following the feedback of antibody test results. It is important to note however that, many of them have taken place in the context of treatment units, where testing was voluntary and where pre- and post-test counselling and support were available. Their results should therefore be treated with caution, since even with adequate support mechanisms, positive test results can significantly increase both depression and anxiety. This could in theory contribute to more chaotic and/or high risk drug use, although empirical evidence on this is lacking (Casadonte *et al.*, 1986).

Testing in the absence of support services is more likely to be harmful than to lead to a reduction in risk behaviour. It has been the impression of one of the authors (Mulleady) that even in the context of a treatment unit people who are antibody positive experience many serious problems in modifying their injecting and sexual behaviour, whereas those who test negative often see this as a 'clean bill of health'. Again, this attitude can result in those who are HIV antibody negative putting themselves at further risk if adequate post-test counselling emphasizing risk reduction is not available. Thus, whilst HIV testing can be an important part of a drug treatment service, it is not a solution to the problem of transmission related behaviour in drug users.

Drug free therapeutic communities can provide many of the

services already discussed, as well as giving syringes to those clients they know are leaving to continue injecting drug use. They have the advantage that their clients are in residence and can therefore develop more sophisticated therapeutic regimes for those who choose to stay.

Syringe Availability

Issues to do with syringe availability are discussed at some length in Stimson's chapter in this volume, where the emphasis was on an analysis of the syringe and needle-exchange scheme set up in Britain in 1987. The evidence suggests that a number of these are not in treatment, and indeed about 60 per cent of clients attending the St. Mary's Drug Dependency Unit exchange scheme are in this group. It is important to recognize though that at any one time the majority of drug users will not be attending a Drug Dependency Unit for treatment (Hartnoll *et al.*, 1985), and indeed we cannot assume that every user will wish to receive treatment if findings from an American study obtain here. Watters *et al.* (1986) found that 53 per cent of ninety-seven drug users contacted in the community in San Francisco would not enter treatment even if it were readily available, and as we have seen (Des Jarlais and Friedman, 1987), drug users in treatment may continue to inject illicit drugs, even if they practise this at a reduced rate. Syringe-exchange schemes therefore exemplify a style of intervention which fulfils clients' needs and may substantially reduce the possibilities for the further transmission of HIV infection. Where available, schemes should be advertised widely, and this includes via local Drug Dependency Units.

Outreach Work

This kind of intervention is far from new and is discussed in detail in the chapter by Hart. Within the context of HIV infection however, outreach work has received increased attention, with the need to reach drug users in the community. Because of the possibility that only the more organized injecting drug users will make use of drug agencies, outreach work may be needed to contact the more chaotic drug user. The success of this kind of intervention relies heavily on the skills of the outreach worker. By its very nature, it can be stressful work to undertake, and adequate support should be available for the workers themselves. It has been suggested that the purpose of outreach work is to inform injecting drug users about existing drug services and to encourage them to use them. However, for those who choose not to avail themselves of these drug services, the outreach worker may be the only source of support with whom they come into contact. This makes the quality of service delivered by the outreach worker all the more important. This in turn will be influenced by a number of factors: the setting for the contact, the people present, what the injecting drug user is willing to listen to, the information they are willing to disclose, the injecting drug user's behaviour in terms of HIV transmission risk, access to local services, and the culture associated with the local drug use scene. In effect, many outreach workers function as 'mobile drug agencies' and, as well as offering information and advice, may provide a limited syringe-exchange service and distribute condoms and spermicide.

Although research into outreach work has so far been primarily concerned to investigate its effectiveness in encouraging injecting drug users to enter treatment (Jackson and Nestin, 1986; Jackson, 1986), in San Francisco a recent study has been undertaken to measure its effect on drug using behaviour in the community (Watters *et al.*, 1986). Bleach was distributed by outreach workers to injecting drug users to be used to sterilize equipment, and whilst only 3 per cent were found to be doing this at the commencement of the programme, six months later 76 per cent reported that they were using the bleach.

A number of programmes have specifically employed users and ex-users as outreach workers, in the belief that these individuals might have higher status and acceptability amongst injecting drug users (McAuliffe *et al.*, 1987; Jackson and Rotkiewicz, 1987). Initiatives like these may also encourage the development of community-based responses to the risks associated with HIV infection.

Liaison with other agencies is an essential component of outreach work. In London, the St. Mary's Drug Dependency Unit works closely with the police in order to advertise the services available. Effective lines of communication also need to exist with other outreach projects in order to ensure that duplication of work and 'territorial' disputes can be kept to a minimum.

Self-Help

Friedman *et al.* (1988) found that injecting drug users were more likely to reduce risk taking behaviour if they saw others taking steps to protect themselves. This highlights the importance of peer group behaviour in influencing risk reduction. It also suggests that self-help activity organized on a community basis can be a useful risk-reduction intervention. A number of self-help groups for drug users already exists. The Junkiebonden in the Netherlands has been in existence for some years, and was formed originally as a pressure group to influence government policy on drug use issues. Similar groups have developed in the United States, for example ADAPT (Association for Drug Abuse Prevention and Treatment).

These groups will probably have a more important impact on injecting drug users' behaviour than any others since they can often communicate directly with drug users themselves. They can also function as sources of information and support. Although a small number of self-help groups for HIV positive injecting drug users and their partners have started throughout the United Kingdom they are in their early stages of development and are often maintained by a few committed individuals. Little systematic research has been carried out so far into their operation.

Self-help groups may prove useful not only for injecting drug users, but also drug workers. The latter may be able to canvass the views of the former about the nature of the services needed locally, the likely take-up of these and the perceived effectiveness of specific interventions. Drug workers would be well advised to encourage and support the development of these groups, by making rooms available for meetings and making their existence known to new clients.

Community Care

According to Miller (1987), people with AIDS who experience the greatest difficulty in adjusting to their situation often have one or more of the following factors in common: poor accommodation, few or poor family ties, low peer acceptance and guilt over past behaviour.

Many of the injecting drug users seen at the St. Mary's Drug Dependency Unit experience some or all of these problems, with housing and financial difficulties being the most common. It is essential that drug workers try to offer practical help in this area. Apart from the benefit to the individual drug user, this can reduce some of the pressure on overburdened hospital wards, since housing problems and the absence of a network of carers in the community can result in longer hospital stays than are strictly necessary for treatment. Many bereaved families of injecting drug users with AIDS have great difficulty in coming to terms with the circumstances of their son or daughter's death. Family support counselling is likely to become increasingly important.

Hospice and respite care is already in short supply. A unit that could provide short-term interim care and accommodation for those in crisis would be useful for injecting drug users. Voluntary organizations too can provide a much needed network of helpers in the community. Tenneriello *et al.* (1987) have described a volunteer network to offer care for people with AIDS. Clients on Methadone maintenance programmes have taken part in this and have proved to be successful members of the team. Some New York clinics offer economic incentives to Methadone clients who do outreach work, helping people with AIDS in the community (Elion, personal communication). Statutory organizations in this country have so far been slow to consider the contribution that users and ex-users could make to their services.

Prevention and Initiation

An individual is often introduced to heroin by his or her peers (Friedman, 1988) and if this drug is taken by injection then it is *likely* that syringes will be shared (Hart, personal communication). So far, we have little knowledge about the extent of recreational or occasional drug use and have little to offer the Amphetamine or Cocaine user in the way of treatment packages. In this situation, education on harm reduction is particularly essential.

As yet we do not have a coordinated school-based education programme on the dangers associated with drug use, and if the subject is addressed it is often left to teachers who have not been given any specific training. Prevention is inevitably better than cure, yet measures taken to reduce harm in drug services, whilst useful, seek to deal with the consequences of what is essentially avoidable behaviour. Therefore, much more effort is required to educate children and young people realistically about what they can and cannot do in terms of risk to self and others. Within this context emphasis must be placed on social skills training. There is now good evidence that prevention programmes based on fear arousal are not very successful in producing behavioural change, particularly if fear is associated with a low probability event or if there is a long time period between the risks associated with drug use and their adverse consequences (*ibid*). If drugs workers can identify specific groups potentially at risk, their efforts are likely to have maximum impact (Sherr, 1987). Where possible, the encouragement of peer group responsibility for continuing prevention must be integrated into teaching.

Training is necessary for staff as well as clients, and a multimedia approach can be used, both with groups and on a one-to-one basis. Outside lecturers, workshops, videos, leaflets, as well as more participatory open days can all be used to good effect here. Good sources of information and high levels of knowledge may be requisites of good preventive drugs work, but generating support and agreement may be the deciding factor in determining whether or not low-risk behaviours are adopted.

Conclusion

In this chapter, we have reviewed a variety of preventive and harm-minimization interventions that can be used with injecting drug users. Although they have been described separately, it is possible to combine interventions to produce discrete packages for individual users. Thus for some individuals, Methadone treatment can be combined with increased availability of injecting equipment as well as participation in a self-help group. Increased access to counselling, medical and family planning care, housing, rehabilitation skills training, advocacy, health education and welfare may all be necessary at some point. Whilst it has not been possible to explore in detail each of these interventions here, all can play a part in facilitating risk reduction and harm-minimization. It is important that services such as these are coordinated at national, regional and district levels if local initiatives to explore new pathways to prevention and risk reduction are to be developed. HIV disease presents a formidable challenge. Are the commitment, political will and resources there to meet it?

References

Bunning, E. C., Verster, A. D. and Gartgers, C. (1987) 'Amsterdam's policy on AIDS and drugs', paper presented at the National Institute on Drug Abuse meeting, Washington, DC, May.

Casadonte, P., Des Jarlais, D. C., Smith, T. S., Novatt, A. and Hemdal, P. (1986) 'Psychological and behavioural impact of learning HTLV III/

LAV antibody test results', paper presented at the International Conference on AIDS, Paris, June.

Connell, P. H. (1975) 'Review of Methadone maintenance schemes', presented at Skandia International Symposia, Stockholm, p 133.

Cox, C. P., Selwyn, P. A., Schoenbaum, E. E., O'Dowd, M. A. and Drucker, E. (1986) 'Psychological and behavioural consequences of HTLV III/LAV antibody testing and notification among intravenous drug abusers in a methadone programme in New York City', paper presented at the International Conference on AIDS, Paris.

Des Jarlais, D. C., Chamberland, M. E. and Yankcovitz, A. R., *et al.* (1984) 'Heterosexual partners: A large risk for AIDS', *Lancet*, 2, pp 1346–7.

Des Jarlais, D. C. and Friedman, S. R. (1987) 'Editorial Review: HIV infection and intravenous drug users: Epidemiology and risk reduction', *AIDS*, 1, pp 67–76.

Friedman, S. R., Des Jarlais, D. C. and Goldsmith, D. S. (1988) 'An overview of current AIDS prevention efforts aimed at intravenous drug users', *Journal of Drug Issues*, submitted for publication.

Goldstein, A. (1971) 'Heroin addiction and the role of methadone in its treatment', *Journal of Psychedic Drugs*, 4, p 177.

Gossop, M. (1987) 'A review of the evidence for methadone as a treatment for narcotic addiction', *Lancet*, 1, pp 812–5.

Hartnoll, R. L., Mitcheson, M. C. and Battersby, M. B. A. *et al.* (1980) 'Evaluation of heroin maintenance in controlled trial', *Archives of General Psychiatry*, 367, pp 877–84.

Hartnoll, R., Mitcheson, M., Lewis, R. and Bryer, S. (1985) 'Estimating the prevalence of opioid dependence', *Lancet*, i, pp 203–5.

Howard, J. and Borges, P. (1970) 'Needle-sharing in the Haight: Some social and psychological functions', *Journal of Health and Social Behaviour*, II, pp 220–30.

Jackson, J. and Nestin, S. (1986) 'Impact of using ex-addict educators to disseminate information on AIDS to intravenous drug users,' presented to be Second International Conference on AIDS, Paris.

Jackson, J. and Rotkiewicz, L. (1987) 'A coupon programme: AIDS education and drug treatment', presented to the Third International Conference on AIDS, Washington, D.C.

McAnliffe, W. E., Doering, S. and Breer, P. *et al.* (1987) 'An evaluation of using ex-addict outreach workers to educate intravenous drug users about AIDS prevention', presented to the Third International Conference on AIDS, Washington, D.C.

Marlink, R.G., Foss, B. and Swift, R. *et al.* (1987) 'High rate of HTLV-III exposure IVDA's from a small sized city and the rate of failure of specialised Methadone maintenance to prevent further drug use', presented at the Third International Conference on AIDS, Washington, D.C.

Miller, D. (1987) HIV counselling: some practical problems and issues. *Journal of the Royal Society of Medicine*, 80, pp 278–80.

Mulleady, G. and Sherr, L. (1988) 'Lifestyle factors in drug users in relation to risks for HIV and AIDS', *AIDS Care*, In press.

Newmeyer, J. A., Feldman, H. W., Biernacki, P. and Walters, J. K. (1988) 'Preventing AIDS contagion among intravenous drug users', *Medical Anthropology*.

Schut, J., File, K. and Wohlmuth, T. W. (1973) 'Implications of patients missing medication visits on a methadone programme', *International Journal of Clinical Pharmacology*, 7, 1, pp 26–31.

Selwyn, P. A., Cox, C. P., Feiner, C., Lipschutz, C. and Cohen, R. (1985) 'Knowledge about AIDS and high risk behaviour among intravenous drug abusers in New York City', paper presented at the annual meeting of the American Public Health Association, Washington, DC, November.

Sherr, L. (1987) 'An evaluation of the UK government health education campaign on AIDS', *Psychology and Health*, 1, pp 61–72.

Tenneriello, L., Poust, B., Callan, M., Gordon, L., Levine, J., Webber, M. and Drucker, E. (1987) 'A hospital-based programme utilizing methadone patients and others to provide support to inner city AIDS patients', paper presented at the Third International Conference on AIDS, Washington, DC, June.

Van Bilsen, H. P. J. G. (1986) 'Heroin addiction, morals re-visited', *Journal of Substance Abuse Treatment*, 3, pp 279–84.

Watters, J. K., Lura, D. M. and Lura, K. W. (1986) *AIDS Prevention and Education Services to Intravenous Drug Users through the Mid-city Consortium to Combat* AIDS: *Administrative Report on the First Six Months.*

Watters, J. K., Newmayer, J. A. and Cheng, Y.-T. (1986) 'Human immunodeficiency virus infection and risk factors among intravenous drug users in San Francisco', paper presented at the American Public Health Association, Las Vegas, October.

Williams, W. V. and Lee, J. (1975) *International Journal of Addictions*, 10, p 599.

13 Marginalized Groups and Health Education About HIV Infection and AIDS

Tina Wiseman

It is now widely accepted that efforts to deal with the threat to public health posed by HIV infection will depend for their success on health education and not on some 'magic bullet' in the form of a drug or vaccine. In order to be effective, however, health education must speak directly to the needs of a wide range of groups. It is therefore as foolish to produce one leaflet to be read by young people, senior citizens and ethnic minority groups alike as it is to imagine that the needs of widely different constituencies can be met using one particular kind of health education involving active learning. What is needed most is diversity of provision — initiatives and strategies that have their starting point in the lived experience of different communities. Without this, it may well be that many people in Britain will 'die of ignorance', despite government exhortations to the contrary.

The House of Commons Select Committee on AIDS (1987) has recently stated that 'the alienation of any sub-group from the rest of society, whether by their own intent or through the attitudes of others, will undermine the public health, since they may not then feel any responsibility to act for the general good, especially in preventing the spread of infection'. Health promoters could do well to heed these words when planning future public health education interventions around HIV and AIDS. Programmes to date have tended to focus either on the so-called high risk groups or on some ill-defined general population. As a result, many people may feel that they are not at risk of infection and, in consequence, may make little effort to protect themselves or others. If attitudes like these are not countered, there is the possibility that HIV will continue to spread, creating a situation in which there may be no alternative other than to rely on a 'magic bullet'. Paying attention to the special needs of sub-groups within the community is, therefore, not a matter of choice, but one of utmost necessity.

In 1984, the World Health organization emphasized the need for active participation in health issues when it offered the following definition of health promotion.

> Health promotion involves the population as a whole in the context of their everyday life, rather than focusing on people at risk for specific diseases . . . is directed towards action on the determinants or causes of health . . . combines diverse, but complementary, methods or approaches . . . aims particularly at effective and concrete public participation . . . Health professionals — particularly in primary health care — have an important role in nurturing and enabling health promotion . . . (WHO, 1984)

There is an important parallel here between the kinds of goals that health educators might aim for (assuming they see their role as concerned with the promotion of health and well-being) and those that have for some time been the concern of development workers in the Third World. In both cases, community participation is taken to be an essential prerequisite for sustainable development. So far few health education initiatives around HIV and AIDS in Britain have required much by way of community participation. Sustained behavioural change is notoriously difficult to bring about and is not likely to occur if people are treated as the passive recipients of health education messages. Health educators working in the field of HIV infection and AIDS should be thinking more in terms of the ways in which the needs of sub-groups within the community can be used as the starting point for their interventions if their work is to bring about lasting changes in behaviour.

Marginalized Groups

Throughout 1986 and 1987 it became increasingly apparent that a significant number of marginalized groups within the community were alienated because little, if any, attention was given to their particular needs. These included (and these terms are used non-exclusively) ethnic minority groups, young people, the physically disabled and those with learning disabilities. The further alienation of some sections of the community is a real possibility, and steps must be taken now to ensure that this trend does not continue. It is worth noting in this respect that the advent of AIDS itself has led to the alienation of certain groups, and despite the health education initiatives that have taken place so far, there is little sign of a diminished trend in this respect.

Perhaps the most obviously marginalized groups in this country are those whose cultural and/or linguistic background marks them out from the 'norm'. Little or no attempt has been made to develop health education strategies that are either culturally acceptable or linguistically appropriate to these various groups, with the result that many of them have as a last resort produced their own leaflets and have organized themselves on a self-help basis. A few attempts have been made to translate existing health education resources into other languages, but scant attention has been paid to the cultural acceptability of information presented in this way. Given the fairly explicit sexual language within which some of the original materials were couched, it is hardly surprising that the translated form may be unacceptable and/or poorly understood in cultural contexts where there may be no corresponding sexually explicit language.

People with learning difficulties have also been overlooked by HIV education so far. Many of the strategies that presently exist assume a fairly high degree of literacy amongst those they seek to involve. For many people, the sheer number of words in a leaflet or poster may be daunting; how much more so must it be for those with learning difficulties? Yet, little attempt has been made to produce information of a more graphic nature. Similarly, discussion of the relevant issues often takes place in unnecessarily complicated medical and scientific terminology when more down-to-earth language can be used. The underlying assumption seems to be that only the verbally 'sophisticated' and the literate are likely to be at risk from HIV infection, and only they need to be provided with opportunities to take the necessary steps to reduce their risk.

Existing health education initiatives have also missed many young people. Some have had too 'boring' a feel to them. Others have used inappropriate terminology. In consequence, some young people have been forced to fall back on their own resources — a situation which is potentially worrying given their probable high degree of sexual activity.

Health Education Interventions

There are a number of ways in which health education about HIV infection and AIDS can take place. Some are more likely than others to be effective in producing desired outcomes. Despite Aggleton and Homans (1987) injunction,

> . . . whilst we appreciate health educators' eagerness to act quickly in the area of AIDS education, we feel it is imperative that people take time to analyze the pressures on them to act in particular ways, (and) to understand how their own and their clients' perceptions of the syndrome may be influenced by cultural and social factors . . .

there is evidence that in the area of HIV education, many of the health education initiatives that have so far taken place have been somewhat narrowly conceived, being immediate rather than carefully considered responses to the present situation.

In recent years, health educators have begun to differentiate between the different styles or models of health education that can be used to help people learn about health issues (Tones, 1981; Ewles and Simnett, 1985; French and Adams, 1986). Within the context of health education about HIV infection and AIDS, Homans and Aggleton (1988) have recently differentiated between information-giving, self-empowerment, community-oriented and socially-transformatory approaches. These set different goals for health education and identify different means by which these can be achieved (see also Aggleton and Homans, 1987). Other health educators have distinguished between what can be called top-down and bottom-up (or grass roots) initiatives (Beattie, 1986). The former tend to focus on issues which policy makers and health educators themselves feel are important. The latter have their origins within the lived experience of the community or sub-groups within it.

If we look at the top-down versus the bottom-up approach in relation to the various models of health education described by Homans and Aggleton (1988), we can see that the information-giving model relies on a top-down approach. Health educators decide what people need to know and make the information available to them through the media. By way of contrast, self-empowerment, community-oriented and socially-transformatory models all rely to varying degrees on a bottom-up approach which involves and encourages community participation. Self-sustaining health awareness

Figure 13.1:

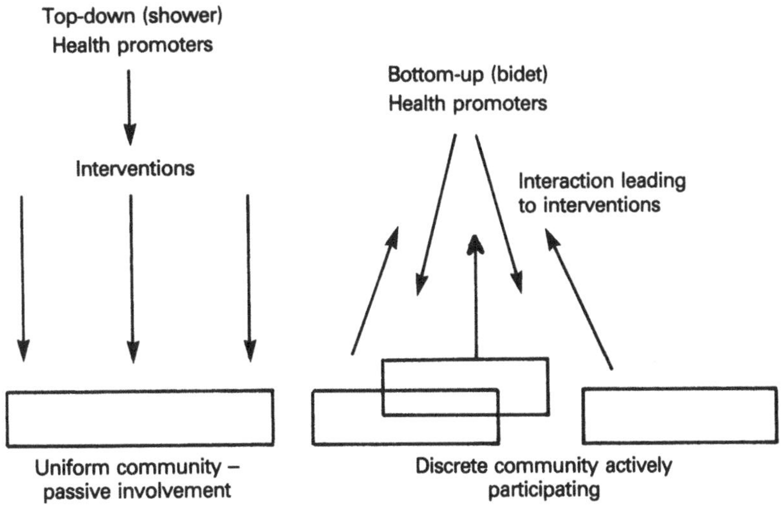

is more likely to emerge from these latter kinds of intervention because the community as a whole, or particular sections of it, is likely to have been actively participating from the very beginning. Information-giving approaches on the other hand, which require that individuals be the passive receptors of health education messages, are unlikely to lead to self-sustaining change. Sad to say, they have been amongst the most widely used strategies in HIV and AIDS education in this country.

A further aid to conceptualizing the processes involved in health education about HIV infection and AIDS can be provided by the distinction between what we can call a 'shower' model of dissemination and a 'bidet' approach (figure 13.1).

The 'shower' approach does not allow for much interaction between health educators and their clients, and the likelihood is that the shower will penetrate the community to a certain extent but will leave some sections of it totally unaffected. Many of the health education resources produced so far seem to be directed towards some kind of 'uniform community' which in reality does not exist. Marginalized groups are therefore not reached and are further alienated by the assumption that they do not have specific needs.

If we contrast this with the 'bidet' model, we can see that a key assumption here is that the community consists of a range of overlapping and separate groups which interact in a variety of ways with health educators and health promoters. This interaction is a vital and necessary process if all members of the community are to be reached and fewer are to be alienated. The styles of interaction that take place will need to be as diverse as the groups themselves.

The Terrence Higgins Trust and Marginalized Groups

Elsewhere, HIV has been described as an 'equal opportunities' virus, and it is becoming increasingly clear that it will infect anyone whose actions put them at risk. This being so, health educators and health promoters can no longer afford the luxury of thinking only in terms of high risk groups. They must turn their attention to high risk behaviours insofar as these may be displayed by anyone in the entire community.

Historically, the Terrence Higgins Trust has directed its efforts towards gay men, a group marginalized by society's inability or reluctance to treat them as equals, and further alienated as a result of AIDS. More recently, attention has also been given to meet the needs of injecting drug users who have suffered from a lack of support at a time when they may be doubly vulnerable. In its work with both of these groups, the Terrence Higgins Trust has attempted to develop a range of interventions that are acceptable to their membership. The alienation of a marginalized group will decrease only if there is sufficient interaction between its members and the health educators and health promoters concerned. It is this process of alienation which we would hope to avoid.

More recently, work has begun with a wider cross-section of marginalized groups. The methods of interaction range from workshops, seminars and counselling, to the formation of support groups and the invitation of speakers. Some groups have been further assisted by the provision of office space, telephone lines and financial resources according to their needs. In this way, groups such as Refugee Action, the National Bureau for Handicapped Children, the Black Community AIDS Team, the Chinese Community Health Care Centre, Greater London Youth Matters and Leicester YMCA have been provided with material and moral support.

The Terrence Higgins Trust has, therefore, demonstrated a flexibility of structure that will allow for a variety of interactions and the absorption of many new support groups. Those working within the Trust have tried to adapt to their expressed needs by listening and providing an arena for discussion. Health interventions are formulated by the groups themselves with members of the Trust acting in a facilitatory role. It is obvious that a wide range of interventions must be considered and current projects range from the funding of videos and drama to advice on translated leaflets and the production of graphic materials.

The Terrence Higgins Trust's interaction with the above groups and others has thus been as varied as the groups themselves. By taking on the role of facilitator/motivator, the Terrence Higgins Trust can enable them to formulate interventions which are appropriate to their needs. In order to encourage active participation, it is vital that health educators and health promoters continue to act primarily in a consultancy role, and assist with appropriate resources only when requested to do so.

The initiative behind any particular intervention must remain with the group concerned if its membership is to participate actively. The role of facilitator is not an easy one to assume; there is always the temptation to 'direct' or 'lead' in some way and thereby take the initiative, but this can be avoided if careful and thorough liaison is maintained throughout. It is some indication of our success in this role that marginalized groups continue to approach us for help, but there is a need for more formal evaluation of the service so far provided.

Conclusions

The Terrence Higgins Trust was conceived by, and grew from within, the gay community and is therefore in a unique position when it comes to dealing with other marginalized groups. This is not to say that there are common problems or even common solutions, but that the methods of interaction may be transferable. Workers at the

Figure 13.2:

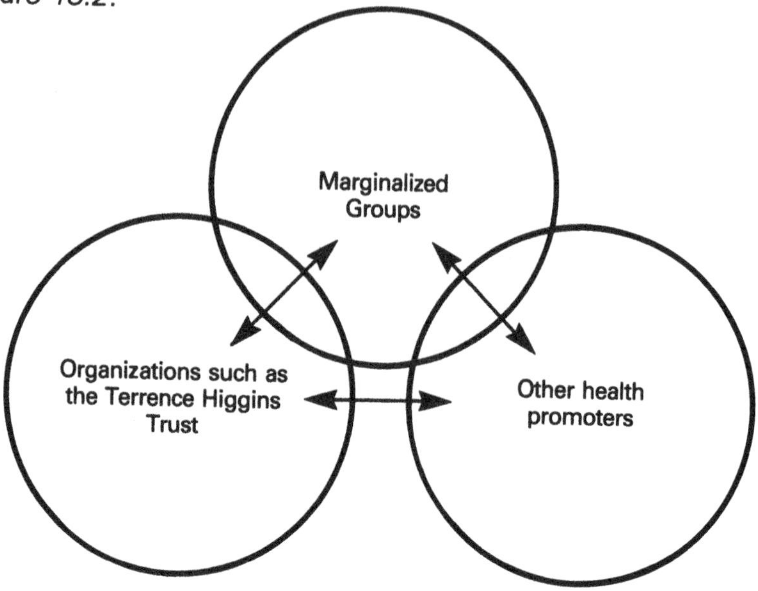

Terrence Higgins Trust have learned from their own experience of coming from an alienated group and more recently, have been able to draw on that experience in forming links with other groups.

A more accurate model of the processes involved in effective health education about HIV might be one which encourages marginalized and alienated groups to interact and learn from each other as well as with health promoters. The success of resulting health interventions will be dependent upon the quality of interaction that led to their development. Poor or inadequate levels of interaction may lead to inappropriate interventions, whilst good interaction will result in interventions that are appropriate and therefore more likely to be effective in encouraging behaviour change (figure 13.2).

In the above figure, the arrows indicate the flow of information in both directions in that we all have something to learn from each other. Similarly, the expressed needs of the various groups are of vital importance and provide the starting point for the development of health interventions. It is only by listening to the needs of others that we can begin to meet these needs. This applies equally as much to different groups within the community as it does to the professional health promoters and the statutory and voluntary bodies they represent. Hopefully, in this way, we will be able to avoid the further alienation of marginalized groups.

The challenge for the future is to demonstrate flexibility and an ability to adapt to the needs of disparate sub-groups within the community rather than just deliver messages. Health educators and health promoters must listen and learn from their prospective clients before they can help them make more rational decisions about their lives. Liaison, networking, learning and adaptation will be crucial factors in the process of promoting active participation. If we can eventually say that the whole community has developed a sustainable health awareness of the issues around HIV and AIDS, then the effort involved will have been more than worthwhile.

Reference

AGGLETON, P. and HOMANS, H. (1987) *Educating about AIDS*, Bristol, National Health Service Training Authority.

BEATTIE, A. (1986) 'Community development for health: From practice to theory', *Radical Health Promotion*, 4, pp 12–18.

EWLES, L. and SIMNETT, I. (1985) *Promoting Health — A Practical Guide to Health Education*, Chichester, Wiley.

FRENCH, J. and ADAMS, L. (1986) 'From analysis to synthesis', *Health Education Journal*, 45, 2, pp 71–4.

HOMANS, H. and AGGLETON, P. J. (1988) 'Health education, HIV infection and AIDS' in AGGLETON, P. and HOMANS, H. (Eds.) *Social Aspects of AIDS*, Lewes, Falmer Press.

Third Report from the Social Services Select Committee (1987) London, HMSO.

TONES, K. (1981) 'Health education, prevention or subversion?', *Journal of the Royal Society of Health*, 3.

WORLD HEALTH ORGANIZATION (1984) *Health Promotion — A Discussion Document on the Concept and Principles*, Supplement to Europe News, 3, Copenhagen, WHO Regional Office for Europe.

14
Evaluating Health Education about AIDS

Peter Aggleton

In Britain about 1700 people have now been diagnosed with AIDS of whom about half have died, and recent estimates suggest that between 50,000 and 100,000 others may already have been infected by the Human Immunodeficiency Virus (HIV), the cause of the syndrome. In the United States, more than 70,000 people have already been diagnosed with AIDS, of whom over half are dead and when official estimates were last published (some two years ago), it was estimated that one-and-a-half to two million Americans could be infected.

As yet there is no cure for AIDS, nor is there a vaccine to protect against infection. Available treatments tend to be limited in their effectiveness and some have debilitating side effects requiring blood transfusions and sometimes the discontinuation of therapy. Whilst a significant number of new advances in treatment are being made, it may be many years before their overall effectiveness can be evaluated.

In this situation, health education has been identified as the most effective means by which to limit the further spread of infection, and there have now been a number of local and national initiatives to achieve this goal. In Britain, much of the early work was carried out by voluntary organizations providing counselling and support for the first people to be affected by AIDS. The Terrence Higgins Trust (THT) is perhaps the best known of these groups. Founded originally by gay men to provide support for other gay men, THT has subsequently expanded its activities to provide services to many other groups. Other organizations which were quick to recognize the need for intervention include the Standing Conference on Drug Abuse (SCODA) and the London Lesbian and Gay Switchboard.

Subsequently, central government, local authorities, district health authorities and voluntary organizations have planned and implemented programmes of health education about HIV infection and AIDS. These have been as diverse as the agencies themselves, and have varied from information-giving exercises in which the emphasis has been on making the facts about AIDS available, often through posters, leaflets, and radio and television advertising, to experiential small group work where the emphasis has been on helping individuals clarify their feelings about the issues that AIDS raises.

Many of the initiatives that have so far taken place have been broadly reactive in nature, being immediate and often well-meaning responses to the challenges posed by AIDS. Because of this, it is not surprising that some have been less successful than others — sometimes being ignored by those they aimed to involve, sometimes arousing strong feelings and hostility when the intention had been to inform and reassure, sometimes fuelling divisive fears and prejudices when the aim had been to enhance social understanding (Craig, 1987).

As we move now to an era in which health education about AIDS can be more systematically planned, implemented and evaluated, it is important to reflect on the strengths and limitations of these early initiatives. By doing this, we may be better able to identify the goals that should be aimed for as well as the most appropriate means by which these might be achieved. But critical evaluation of this kind presupposes a willingness on the part of health educators to stand back (albeit momentarily) from the work with which they are most immediately involved. For some, especially those who are involved in the ongoing support and counselling of people with HIV infection and/or AIDS, this may be no easy thing to do. At a personal level, there may be feelings of guilt to contend with — actions such as these may be felt to be letting down those who are most in need. There is also the possibility that a concern to evaluate AIDS education may be construed by others as prevarication and a desire to academicize when what is needed most is purposeful and practical intervention.

However, without this kind of critical evaluation, health education about AIDS is likely to be ill conceived. Health educators who fail to evaluate the activities with which they are involved are unlikely to learn from their own successes and mistakes, as well as those of others. They may also allow their enthusiasm for a particular style of health education to cloud a more rational assessment of its overall effectiveness. Finally, they may run the risk of rediscovering what others already know — the limitations of particular kinds of health education in achieving certain goals.

In this chapter, an attempt will be made to identify the options open to health educators as they set about critically evaluating their own work and that of others. In order to do this, it will first be necessary to consider some of the different ways in which health education about AIDS can take place. Only then will it be possible to identify appropriate evaluation strategies.

Health Education about AIDS

People can learn about health and health-related issues in many different ways. These different styles of health education (or models of health education as they are increasingly called) differ from one another both in terms of the goals they set for health education as well as the means by which these can be achieved (Ewles and Simnett, 1985; French and Adams, 1986; Aggleton and Homans, 1987). By far the most familiar model of health education is the information-giving model. This aims to bring about changes in behaviour by providing people with the 'facts' about a particular issue — be it smoking, alcohol consumption, diet or HIV infection.

Other models of health education have different goals. Some may aim to enhance self-empowerment — the ability to act more rationally and purposefully in the pursuit of self determined interests. Others may seek to encourage greater community involvement in health issues. Yet others may aim to bring about far-reaching social change. On the whole, these alternative models of health education advocate a more participatory approach to learning about health and health-related issues.

Moreover, they share a number of features in common. First, they suggest that people value the opportunity to explore for themselves and with others the 'facts' about a particular health issue. Second, they suggest that feelings, attitudes and emotional responses can interfere with the ability to think and behave rationally. Third, they suggest that far from being passive receivers of information, people actively work on the health messages they encounter, reinterpreting these in the light of past experience, and according to present needs.

Information Giving and Health Education about AIDS

According to the information-giving model, the principal aim of health education about AIDS should be to provide people with the

Table 14.1 Four models of health education

	Goals of the model	**Means of achieving these**
INFORMATION-GIVING MODEL	To reduce the incidence of disease by bringing about changes in individual behaviour.	'Facts' and information on health and disease are presented to or 'given' to people by the health educator.
SELF-EMPOWERMENT MODEL	To reduce the incidence of illness and disease by enhancing people's ability to act rationally rather than on the basis of emotions and feelings.	Participatory learning, group work and self-exploration to help clients identify the choices they can make.
COMMUNITY-ORIENTED MODEL	To enhance health by bringing about community change through collective action.	Participatory learning and group work around shared experiences, leading to the identification of collective needs and planning to meet these.
SOCIALLY TRANSFORMATORY MODEL	To enhance health by bringing about far reaching social change throughout society.	Participatory learning and group work around shared experiences to enable the development of a critical awareness of the societal factors affecting health and well-being. These same techniques are then used to help groups act to change the conditions that limit health and well-being.

facts about HIV, its modes of transmission and its possible consequences. They will then be able to modify their behaviour so as not to put themselves and others at risk of infection. This particular style of health education has been widely used in a variety of national and local initiatives. It operates from the assumption that people are rational decision makers and seeks to use information-giving as a means by which to bring about behavioural change.

In Britain, the government's public information campaign launched in spring 1986 used exactly this kind of strategy to inform people about the ways in which the virus is transmitted and the steps that can be taken to reduce the risk of infection. Initially, full page advertisements in the national press were used to provide the facts about HIV and its modes of transmission. Subsequently, cinema, television and radio advertising to enhance public awareness about AIDS and, in early 1987, a leaflet entitled 'AIDS: Don't Die of Ignorance' was distributed to over 20 million households. Autumn of 1987 saw the next stage of the campaign, with the emphasis shifting to the risks associated with injecting drug use, and in February 1988 (after responsibility for this kind of health education moved from the Department of Health and Social Security to the newly-constituted Health Education Authority), the most recent wave of intervention was announced. This time the emphasis was to be on heterosexuals, particularly young heterosexuals, whose sexual behaviour might put them at risk.

Health education like this has, of course, been paralleled by local interventions in schools and colleges, adult and community education, and health and social services provision. Some institutions have organized conferences and meetings where information about AIDS has been given by physicians, health education officers and other experts. Others have shown films and videos or used posters and leaflets to inform people about the risks of infection.

As a result, and within a remarkably short period of time, the information-giving model has become the dominant paradigm within which health education about HIV infection and AIDS takes place in Britain.

Alternative Approaches to Health Education about AIDS

There are, of course, alternatives to the strategy outlined above. Some of these have sought to operate within an information-giving framework but have tried to personalize their messages and make them available via the social groups of which individuals are a part (Gatherer *et al.*, 1979). The success of the Los Angeles 'LA Cares . . . like a Mother' campaign and the San Francisco 'Stop AIDS' campaign has been attributed to the efforts both of these made to personalize health education messages and to make these available via the community structures of which targetted individuals were already a part (Aggleton and Homans, 1987 and 1988; Silin, 1987).

Other strategies have attempted to complement public information initiatives by providing opportunities for people to explore with others what they already know and feel about HIV infection and AIDS. This alternative paradigm, which generally has a more participatory emphasis, is of course far from new. For years, professional health educators have known that the information they make available is not received uniformly by those at whom it is directed. How people process health education information is dependent amongst other things on their mood and motivation, their past learning, their interest in the issue, and its perceived relevance (Phillips, 1988). Lay or popular beliefs about health also have a role to play in mediating the impact of official health education messages (Helman, 1978; Fitzpatrick, 1984, Herzlich and Pierret, 1986; Aggleton and Homans, 1987). People actively work on the information to which they are exposed, reinterpreting it in the light of their past experience and in accordance with their present needs. Health educators have also been aware for some time that the link between knowledge and behaviour is far from direct. The groups to which people belong, personal perceptions of risk and feelings of personal efficacy may be critical in determining the actions taken in response to health education initiatives.

All of this suggests that health education which provides opportunities for people to clarify what they *know* about an issue, to distinguish this from what they *feel* about the same issue, and then to consider the intrapersonal, interpersonal and social barriers to behavioural change will be important. This emphasis underpins many health education initiatives that have self-empowerment as their goal. It has also been the impetus behind a number of community-oriented interventions as well as those that have adopted a more socially-transformatory approach.

Health education with an emphasis on *self-empowerment* aims to encourage people to develop skills, understandings and awareness so that they can act on the basis of rational thought rather than irrational feelings (Aggleton and Homans, 1987). Group work, problem-solving techniques and client-centred counselling are often used to enable individuals to identify the extent to which emotions and attitudes may block an ability to act rationally and sensibly. This particular emphasis has underpinned a variety of health education initiatives funded by local authorities, health authorities and the voluntary sector. In these contexts, re-evaluation co-counselling, assertiveness training, sexuality awareness workshops and other techniques have been widely used to educate about HIV and AIDS.

Whilst self-empowerment strategies can be valuable in identifying the untapped potential that lies within people, and while in some circumstances they can be sufficient to allow people to begin to make safer health choices, they suffer from a number of deficiencies. Most of these stem from their focus on the individual. Thus someone who has been through a self-awareness workshop or an assertiveness training course may *feel* more powerful at the end of it, but these feelings often disappear once the situation that led to the original feeling of powerlessness is re-encountered.

In consequence, some health educators have abandoned strategies like these in favour of more collective and community based approaches. Community-oriented styles of health education reject the idea that the individual is responsible for his or her own health and suggest that people should act collectively to identify and satisfy their health needs. Within the context of health education about AIDS, the actions of organizations such as the Terrence Higgins Trust and local Body Positive groups have often had this kind of focus. Founded originally by gay men to provide education, counselling and support for those affected by HIV infection, the community-based initiatives of the Terrence Higgins Trust have been widely identified as critical in bringing about substantial behavioural change amongst gay men living in London and elsewhere. Other groups that have adopted this particular strategy include a number of voluntary organizations providing counselling, advice and services for injecting drug users and prostitutes.

Community-oriented health education, however, is likely to encounter various obstacles to the attainment of its goals. In particular, it may lead to the identification of resource issues that need to be addressed, political interventions that need to be made, and images and understandings that need to be challenged. In short, it may cause those involved to question the conservatism of strategies which do little to tackle pervasive inequalities of power in society (Adams, 1985; Aggleton and Homans, 1988).

This can be the start of a more socially transformatory approach — one which seeks to enhance health and well-being by bringing about far reaching social change. So far, relatively few initiatives of this kind have taken place within AIDS education, although the beginnings of the style of intervention can be seen in the actions of groups in the United States committed to direct action in order to achieve their goals. Perhaps the best known of these is ACTUP (AIDS Coalition to Unleash Power) which in recent months has been influential in pressurizing the New York State Public Health Council to expedite the development of drug therapies and in questioning the composition and findings of the recent Presidential Commission on HIV infection and AIDS (Zwickler, 1988). Here in Britain there are continuing discussions within groups such as Frontliners (a London-based group of people with AIDS) about the adequacy of strategies which fail to challenge publically the priorities central government has set with respect to research and health education.

Evaluating Health Education about AIDS

Having identified some of the main frameworks within which health education about HIV and AIDS can take place, it is appropriate to consider the strategies that can be used to evaluate the effectiveness of particular kinds of intervention. In doing this, it is essential to bear in mind that different styles of health education may need to be evaluated differently according to the goals they set and the means they advocate to achieve these. Education about HIV and AIDS should therefore be evaluated using criteria specific to the paradigm (or paradigms) within which it takes place. There can therefore be no universal set of criteria against which every initiative can be judged.

Nevertheless, there are a number of key principles that should be borne in mind no matter what style of education is being considered. In this chapter, particular attention will be given to two rather different sets of concerns: the issue of *what* should be evaluated, and the issue of *who* should do the evaluating. In examining the first of these concerns, a critical distinction will be made between outcome and process evaluation. In looking at the second, the issue of insider as opposed to outsider evaluation will be addressed.

The distinction between outcome and process evaluation is by no means new and relates to the contrast that is sometimes drawn between the goals of a particular educational venture and the means by which these are achieved. Given widespread concern that health education about AIDS and HIV should have observable and beneficial consequences, and given the emphasis there has so far been on information-giving, it is not surprising to find that most studies so far have focused on outcome rather than process evaluation. This can be seen most graphically in the recent evaluation of the British government's public information campaigns carried out for the Department of Health and Social Security (DHSS, 1987), but it is also to be found in recent evaluations of more local initiatives.

Outcome Evaluation

Many different kinds of outcome can be associated with health education about AIDS and HIV. Some of these can be *cognitive* in nature, relating perhaps to greater knowledge about the virus and its modes of transmission. Others may be *attitudinal*, relating more closely to the feelings people have about AIDS and those affected by it. Yet others may be *behavioural*, operating either at the level of the individual, or the group, or the community. Contrary to popular belief, there is no reason to assume that change in any one of these three different kinds of outcome will necessarily be mirrored by change in any of the others. Thus an enhanced awareness of the ways in which HIV is (and is not) transmitted will not necessarily be accompanied by behavioural or attitudinal change.

An important distinction can be drawn between the intended outcomes of health education and other less intended consequences (Eisner, 1979). For example, while an enhanced level of awareness about the steps that can be taken to guard against infection might be an intended consequence of some information-giving initiatives, a parallel rise in social anxiety might not be. Recent research by Hastings and Scott (1987) evaluating the Department of Health and Social Security's information-giving initiatives throughout 1986 and 1987 suggests that to some extent this did indeed take place, being an unintended by-product of a campaign whose stated purpose had been to:

> warn the whole population about the potential dangers and to *reassure people* who might have been alarmed by sensational or inaccurate reporting in the press. (DHSS AIDS Unit, 1988, emphasis added)

In the case of information-giving styles of health education, outcome evaluation often focuses on changes in levels of knowledge. It may also enquire into the behavioural and attitudinal correlates of cognitive change, be these intended or otherwise. This particular approach to evaluation is often carried out using a case-control design, with an assessment of knowledge levels being undertaken before and after the health education programme. On other occasions, when a control group cannot be created, as is often the case in mass education initiatives, efforts may be made to monitor changes in knowledge over time. This strategy was adopted in the evaluation of the 1986–1987 British public information campaign referred to above. Findings from this suggest that over the timescale concerned, there were major increases in knowledge about transmission and risk reduction. However, amongst the heterosexual population at least there were few reported changes in sexual behaviour (DHSS, 1987; Hornik, 1987).

In the case of health education with a commitment to self-empowerment, outcome evaluation is likely to have the individual, rather than the group, as its unit of analysis. Of particular concern will be the extent to which he or she feels more powerful after participating in the health education programme. It may also be important to enquire into whether the individual feels able to act more rationally and without unnecessary emotion and prejudice in key situations. Within the context of health education about AIDS and HIV, these may include situations in which the prejudice and irrationality of others is challenged, those in which decisions are made about the adoption of safer sexual practices and those where the individual comes to grips with his or her own feelings about death and bereavement. In evaluating the outcomes of this particular kind of health education, attention may also be focused on the extent to which a sense of self-empowerment persists across different contexts and situations. The views of others who come into contact with the newly empowered individual may need to be sought in order to do this.

With respect to community-oriented initiatives, the kind of outcomes to be looked for will include the extent to which community awareness has been enhanced, the extent to which there has been genuine community involvement in the health education programme, and the degree to which collective involvement in community issues is self-sustaining. It may also be important to examine the kinds of community structures that come into being during and after the health education intervention itself. Particular attention can be given to the form these take, the division of labour within them, their openness or otherwise, and the ways in which they manage change.

Outcome evaluation of health education with a commitment to social transformation is likely to enquire into the extent to which personal, fleeting and sporadic critical insights have become more public, more systematic and more collectively shared. It is also likely to focus on changes in popular understandings of HIV and AIDS, shifts in popular perceptions of disease and disability, and changes in the evaluation of categories of person most likely to be affected. Particular attention may also be given to examining how successfully homophobia, heterosexism and racism have been challenged in the intellectual and cultural agendas that surround AIDS (see the chapters by Weeks and Watney elsewhere in this book). Issues of resource allocation are also likely to be addressed in evaluating the effectiveness of health education within this paradigm, and efforts may be made to assess the extent to which funding priorities have altered so as to benefit the development of more adequate forms of health and social service provision.

Process Evaluation

Health education evaluation requires more than a consideration of outcomes. If we are to learn why some interventions were successful and others less so, we need to understand *how* and *why* they worked. This requires a consideration of the processes involved as well as their consequences (Elliott, 1979). Process evaluation aims to identify how certain outcomes were achieved by illuminating the gap between the health educators' intentions and the measured effects of a programme of intervention. Its focus is often on the transactions that take place between educators and their clients, between clients and their broader social networks, and between clients and the issues they are invited to engage with (Stake, 1967). As such, it is as likely to emphasize the 'learning milieu' and the competing interests that operate within it as the outcomes of education themselves (Parlett and Hamilton, 1972).

Process evaluation is likely to seek information from a variety of sources in an effort to identify competing perspectives on the processes involved in education (Simons, 1981). In the context of health education about AIDS, it will involve data collection from those who were directly targeted by, or who directly participated in, a particular initiative as well as those subsequently influenced by members of this primary group. The focus should therefore be both on the transactions that take place within health education and those that later take place as others come into contact with those who have been educated. Health educators wishing to evaluate their work in this way may find it helpful to consider the kinds of data that should be collected in four critical contexts or environments — the professional context, the peer group context, the personal context and (for some) the parental context (Aggleton and Homans, 1987).

In evaluating the processes associated with an information-giving model of health education about AIDS, it will be important to focus first on the nature of the relationships established between the health educator and her 'audience'. Additional data may need to be collected however on the timing, frequency and context of the communication itself. By doing this, it may be possible to identify some of the intrapersonal and interpersonal factors influencing the way in which health education about AIDS is taken up and used. The interaction between the source of health education messages, their content, the manner in which they are communicated, lay beliefs about health, cultural codes and meanings, and broader structural determinants will also need to be explored if insight is to be gained into how the effects of particular initiatives have been brought about.

Beyond the immediate situation in which health education took place, it will be important to examine the kinds of ongoing relationships established between those who have been educated using this particular approach and others with whom they come into contact. In doing this, it will be important to ask in what ways the structure of these latter relationships reproduces the power hierarchy implicit in the original information-giving encounter or whether there can be variable outcomes here.

Process evaluation associated with of a self-empowerment approach to education about AIDS on the other hand will pay close attention to the nature of the participatory learning that took place. In particular, it will seek to identify the processes that were most effective in bringing about a sense of enhanced personal efficacy. In order to do this, it will be important to focus on the role of facilitator as well as the nature of the activities with which participants were invited to engage.

It will also be important to examine the kind of relationships which newly empowered individuals seek to establish with others. In order to do this, evaluators may find themselves asking in what kinds of ways and through what kinds of processes can an enhanced sense of self-empowerment show itself? How can the changes that accompany self-empowerment be recognized by others? It will also be useful to identify the institutional practices that are most likely to support newly empowered individuals in their actions and the kinds of resistances and countervailing forces that are most influential in causing a sense of enhanced personal efficacy to dissipate. Moreover, it will be significant to examine the extent to which self-empowerment within, say, the professional context can generalize to other more personal spheres of interaction.

When it comes to evaluating the processes associated with a community-oriented style of health education, it will be necessary to examine the mechanisms by which community priorities were first identified. In doing this, it may be useful to consider the role the health educator played in this, the extent to which a top-down or a grass-roots strategy was employed (Beattie, 1986), and the tensions that arose throughout this process. It will also be important to consider how representative were the needs identified of the broad spread of community interests, and how shared were the processes of planning that took place.

Beyond the immediate context of the health education initiative, process evaluation within a community-oriented paradigm may need to enquire into the kinds of ongoing relationships that came to be established between the focus of the health education activity and other community structures. Questions which may be asked here include those that seek to elucidate the kinds of links that were made with existing community health initiatives. They may also try to identify how these relationships changed over time, and in response to what combination of forces. Moreover, what were the mechanisms that led some of these relationships to be self-sustaining, and what were the processes that led to conflict and tension?

Finally, when it comes to an evaluation of socially transformatory health education about AIDS, it will be vital to identify the processes that were most effective in tapping and making available as an educational resource the critical insights of different individuals and groups. Similarly, it will be important to examine the kinds of participatory learning that were most effective in collectivizing and systematizing these perceptions and the strategies that were most successful in influencing decision-makers and others controlling access to resources. Associated issues that may need to be addressed include the kinds of alliances that best facilitate social change and the kinds of resistances that might be expected along the way to achieving this.

In looking beyond the immediate context in which this last style of health education takes place, evaluators may find it helpful to focus on those processes that brought about social change within the services provided by the health service, local authorities, central government and agencies working within the voluntary sector. Particular attention may be given here to the kinds of alliances within, and between, these different aspects of service provision that were most successful in bringing about greater social justice.

Who Should Evaluate?

Reference was made earlier to the enthusiasm with which particular styles of health education are often embraced by their adherents. This cautions against an approach to evaluation which relies on insider perspectives alone, since these may be seriously distorted by the evaluator's desire (conscious or otherwise) to show their work in a favourable light. Nevertheless, a sensitivity to the goals associated with different models of health education is essential if evaluation is to do justice to the interventions that have taken place. Because of this, external evaluators working in the area of AIDS education may need a sensitivity, a wholeheartedness and a broadmindedness that is not always encountered amongst their counterparts working in more mainstream health education. In particular, they will have to consider carefully the extent to which they genuinely understand the goals that can be aimed for via different models of health education. Many will also need to develop the skills of insight needed to identify the innovative but sometimes unintended outcomes that can follow from different styles of intervention.

Moreover, in the field of health education about AIDS, the politics of evaluation are likely to be particularly complex, since not only are evaluators likely to be faced with the demand that an initiative should be successful in limiting the potential spread of infection, they may also have to contend with pressures that it should be evaluated in accordance with the extent to which it does so within a particular moral or social framework.

In this latter respect, there may be an additional set of dilemmas to contend with, relating to the qualities of those best suited to evaluate health education about AIDS and HIV. There is no reason to suppose *a priori* that those experienced in evaluating mainstream health education will necessarily have the commitment and sensitivity to work effectively in an area which raises complex issues to do with race, sexuality and the rights of minority communities. Efforts to counter racism, homophobia and heterosexism, for example, which have been the intent of some health education projects in this field, may arouse strong emotions in those of a conservative or even a liberal persuasion. Similarly, efforts to link health education about AIDS to the promotion of monogamy and so-called traditional family values may run contrary to the persuasions of evaluators who seek to temper their concern for expediency with a respect for the many ways in which consensual sexual relationships can take place. These are issues which will require sustained debate and careful working through. Certainly, it will be important for evaluators to make clear their own stance on these and other issues when they begin their work.

Finally, there is the issue of holism to be addressed. Given the diversity of ways in which health education about AIDS can take place and given the various goals that different models of health education seek to attain, it is vital that evaluators adopt a multi-faceted approach. At the present time, there is no place for efforts to privilege one particular evaluative strategy above others — yet sadly there are some signs that this is already taking place, with an evaluation of anticipated outcomes taking precedent over an evaluation of less intended consequences and the means by which these were attained.

To some extent this situation can be accounted for by the speed with which education to do with HIV infection has been rendered accountable to the institutional imperatives of medicine and its allied practices. As Frankenberg and Watney identify (from very different perspectives) elsewhere in this book, the British response to health education about HIV infection and AIDS can be characterized by an initial indifference followed by a sustained effort to incorporate this activity within the institutional framework, and according to the disciplinary imperatives, of the Department of Health and Social Security. Only after the quasi-autonomous Health Education Council had been reconstituted as the Health Education Authority (with clearer lines of accountability to central government) was it considered appropriate to devolve health education about AIDS to this specialist body.

Elsewhere, as Davies' chapter makes clear, the priorities and scientific and medical enquiry still dominate the research agendas to which social researchers and educationalists are expected to subscribe. All this bodes ill for the future. For scientists and physicians are (with one or two exceptions) not well versed in the intricacies of communication and media theory, the psychology of interpersonal processes or, more importantly for the discussion here, *educational evaluation*. Few have undertaken postgraduate study or training in these fields, and the undergraduate curricula they follow are not renowned for the time they allocate to issues of psychological, sociological, cultural and educational concern.

This situation is further complicated by the concerns of New Right politicians and opinion makers to capture health education about HIV infection and AIDS for the reconstruction of a 'traditional' morality that seeks to privilege above all other forms of sexual expression those that are narrowly focused upon procreative and penetrative vaginal intercourse within the context of exclusive and life-long monogamous relationships (see the chapters by Patton, Grover and Watney elsewhere in this book).

In this kind of situation, the temptation may be for agenda setters and decision-makers to fall back on styles of evaluation that are severely limiting. These are not infrequently positivist in the assumptions they make and focused narrowly on the relationship between objectives and measured outcomes. As such, they are unlikely to shed much light on three key sets of factors — learning processes, the unintended consequences of educational interventions and the reasons why particular styles of education may succeed or fail. As Stenhouse (1975) has put it, 'The crucial criticism of the objectives model is that it assesses without explaining . . . hence the developer of the curriculum cannot learn from it'.

An allied problem can arise if only those outcomes and processes that are of scientific or medical interest come to be seen as worthy of investigation. Important psychological, social, political and cultural processes which may reveal why certain outcomes were achieved and others were not may thereby be ignored. It is essential, therefore, that health educators do not abdicate responsibility in this field. In the coming months, they will have a key role to play in educating scientists, doctors and policy makers about the processes of education itself. If they fail in this task or leave it to others, of one thing we can be sure, there will have been many lost opportunities and many more unnecessary deaths.

References

Adams, L. (1985) 'Health education: In whose interest?', unpublished MA dissertation, University of London, Kings College.

Adrien, A. and Carsley, J. (1987) 'A campaign to promote safe sexual practices in the Montreal homosexual population — Quebec', *Canada Diseases Weekly Report*, 13, 3, pp 9–12.

Aggleton, P. and Homans, H. (1987) *Educating about AIDS — A Discussion Document for Community Physicians, Health Education Officers, Health Advisers and Others with a Responsibility for Education about AIDS*, Bristol, Bristol National Health Service Training Authority.

Aggleton, P. and Homans, H. (1988) 'Health education, HIV infection and AIDS' in Aggleton, P. and Homans, H. (Eds.) *Social Aspects of AIDS*, Lewes, Falmer Press.

Aggleton, P. J., Homans, H. Mojsa, J., Watney, S. and Watson, S. (1988) *AIDS: Scientific and Social Issues*, Edinburgh, Churchill–Livingstone.

Beattie, A. (1986) 'Community development for health: From practice to theory', *Radical Health Promotion*, 4, pp 12–18.

Craig, M. (1987) *Report on the AIDS Training Project*, Bristol, Bristol National Health Service Training Authority.

DHSS (1987) *AIDS: Monitoring Responses to the Public Education Campaign*

February 1986–February 1987, London, HMSO.
DHSS AIDS Unit (1988) *AIDS — the UK Response*, London, DHSS.
Eisner, E. W. (1979) *The Educational Imagination: On the Design and Evaluation of School Programmes*, New York, Macmillan.
Elliott, J. (1979) 'Curriculum evaluation and the classroom', paper prepared for the DES Regional Course on Curriculum and Administration. Cambridge Institute of Education, mimeo.
Ewles, L. and Simnett, I. (1985) *Promoting Health — a Guide to Health Education*, Chichester, Wiley.
Fitzpatrick, R. (1984) 'Lay concepts of illness' in Fitzpatrick, R. *et al.* (Eds.) *The Experience of Illness*, London, Tavistock.
French, J. and Adams, L. (1986) 'From analysis to synthesis', *Health Education Journal*, 45, 2, pp 71–4.
Gatherer, A. *et al.* (1979) *Is Health Education Effective?*, London, Health Education Council.
Hastings, G. and Scott, A. (1987) 'AIDS publicity: Pointers to development', *Health Education Journal*, 46, 2, pp 58–9.
Helman, C. (1978) '"Feed a cold, starve a fever": Folk models of infection in an English suburban community and their relation to medical treatment', *Culture, Medicine and Psychiatry*, 2, pp 107–37.
Herzlich, C. and Pierret, J. (1986) 'Illness: From causes to meaning', in Currer, C. and Stacey, M. (Eds.) *Concepts of Health, Illness and Disease*, Leamington Spa, Berg.
Hornik, R. (1987) 'Evaluation strategies: Comparable findings from Australia, Sweden and the United Kingdom', *AIDS Health Promotion Exchange*, 1, pp 9–11.
Jacobs, R. (1987) 'A model for AIDS prevention', *Focus*.
Parlett, M. and Hamilton, D. (1972) *Evaluation as Illumination: A New Approach to the Study of Innovative Programmes*, Occasional paper 9, Centre for Research in the Educational Sciences, University of Edinburgh.
Phillips, K. (1988) 'Strategies against AIDS', *The Psychologist*, 1, 2, pp 46–7.
Silin, J. (1987) 'Dangerous knowledge', *Christopher Street*, 113, pp 34–40.
Simons, H. (1981) 'Process evaluation in schools' in Lacey, C. and Lawton, D. (Eds.) *Issues in Evaluation and Accountability*, London, Methuen.
Stake, R. (1967) 'The countenance of educational evaluation', *Teachers College Record*, 68, 7.
Stenhouse, L. (1985) *An Introduction to Curriculum Research and Development*, London, Heinemann.
Zwickler, P. (1988) 'State panel hears activists', *New York Native*, 246, p 11.

15
Resistance and the Erotic

Cindy Patton

In the past year there has been a surge of interest in the topic of AIDS.[1] Yet the history of resistance to the political crisis surrounding AIDS is in danger of being lost to a revised history that counts only the actions and concerns of the professionals who have taken up AIDS as an issue. The instant experts of 1987 — well-intentioned and intelligent people with the power to convey information and set policy — are not largely the true experts, those who have been involved in sorting out the wide-ranging effects of AIDS since the epidemic began. It is critical that the experience of the gay community in AIDS organizing be understood: the strategies employed before 1985 or so grew out of gay liberation and feminist theory. It is also axiomatic that those most affected — the gay, injecting drug user, black, Hispanic and sex work communities — be listened to when we set new strategies and draw new lines of resistance.

Claiming Safer Sex History

At the 1987 lesbian and gay health conference in Los Angeles, many long-time AIDS activists were surprised by the extent to which safer sex education had become the province of high level professionals. The fact that safer sex organizing began and is highly successful as a grassroots, community effort seemed to be forgotten. It was as if the professionals had invented safer sex. Although professional health and sex educators have made important contributions to AIDS education, their work came long after a community under siege had mobilized to protect itself.

Mainstream accounts of AIDS provide even less reference to the roots of safer sex organizing in the gay community. Heterosexuals — and even gay people only beginning to confront AIDS — express panic about how to make appropriate and satisfying changes in their sex lives, as if no one had done this before them. It is a mark of the intransigence of homophobia that few look to the urban gay communities for advice, communities which have an infrastructure and a track record of highly successful behaviour change.

The overprofessionalization of safer sex organizing, and the lack of historical insight by professionals, has a direct effect on the style of education for gay men and heterosexuals. Many lesbians and gay men just laughed at the silly 'say "NO" to sex' pronouncements of Reagan officials, but there is a hidden price to this smugness. Lost are the innovative projects in cities like Houston, Los Angeles, Chicago, New York and Boston, that worked within the existing cultural structure of the gay male community to educate and affect sexual norms.[2] In public, most health educators are no longer willing to take social risks in order to promote greater sexual safety.

It is essential that those concerned with the broader implications of AIDS understand the history of the gay community's safer sex organizing. These successes are derived from gay activists, not from public health professionals who came late and reluctantly into the health crisis. If we embrace a revised history in which professionals imagine that they conjured safer sex out of formulas and studies, we will become even more dependent on a medical establishment that is so callous towards women's, gay, and minority health concerns.

'How to Have Sex in an Epidemic'

Safer sex organizing began almost as soon as AIDS was recognized, and organizing within the gay community originated in opposition to pronouncements of doctors largely ignorant about gay male sexuality. Their advice assumed that all gay men did the same thing, or that any individual gay man did only one set of practices — for example, that a man was exclusively the object of anal sex, or only sucked cock (the stereotypical 'queer' activities, with, no doubt 'real men' on the other end of the bargain).

Badly-designed studies and homophobia combined to create a flurry of nonsensical, insulting advice. At the 1985 International AIDS Conference in Atlanta, for example, a Centers for Disease Control (CDC) official proposed that all gay men take the then-new (and not extensively tested) HTLV-III antibody test (hereafter called by its current name, HIV antibody test). He further suggested that gay men should only have sex with men of the same antibody status, as if gay male culture is little more than a giant dating service. This advice was quickly seen as dehumanizing and not useful because it did not promote safer sex, but renewed advice of this type has been seen as reasonable within the heterosexual community of late. Gay men quickly came up with their own advice, and coined the term 'safer sex'. Sorting through the same data, and adding knowledge about other sexually transmitted diseases (STDs) among gay men, activists thereby created safer sex guidelines even before the virus was identified.

By May 1983 so much material about safer sex had been distributed through clinics and in the gay press that a group of men — including men with AIDS — produced a 40-page pamphlet called *How to Have Sex in an Epidemic*. This still stands as one of the best and most comprehensive explanations of transmission models, safer sex and psychosocial guidelines for effecting risk reduction. Most importantly, it proposes a plan for change that is couched in terms of a community resistance.

Considerable controversy surrounded the publication of this booklet, foreshadowing the political struggles which were later to engage sex educators and community activists. Two principal criticisms of the booklet emerged: some thought the only sound advice was to advocate celibacy, while others thought it irresponsible to offer specific advice until there was certainty about the transmission and cause of the disease. The celibacy solution is still promoted by the right, in tandem with the idea that gay sex is intrinsically hazardous. Their political agenda of indicting all sex outside monogamous marriage focuses attention on intercourse; and obscures the pleasures of non-penetrative sexual activities for gay and straight alike. In addition to right-wing homophobes, some politically-conscious AIDS educators do advocate celibacy for gay and straight youth, arguing that they need time to gain competence in safer sex technical and negotiation skills.

Responsible Advice? or the Responsibility to Advise?

The second objection — when is it responsible to give advice? — has been played out in more insidious ways. The inability to decide specifically what is safe and unsafe has prevented many groups from recommending what is safe in broad terms. Counsellors and safer sex educators, especially doctors, are often unwilling to say that anything is safe. They are afraid someone will acquire HIV infection while taking their advice. This mixed message leaves people confused about what is unsafe and gives an underlying impression that everything is equally unsafe. This is a troublesome misperception; studies of behavioural changes among gay men showed that those made early in the epidemic were based on perceived need to change or reduce the least favourite activity, not the most dangerous activity. Ironically, a different attitude is now taken in some youth education programmes: a New York City Lesbian and Gay Centre Youth Project advocates telling youths that unprotected anal and vaginal sex are absolutely unsafe, and if young people feel they can give up only one thing, using condoms or refraining from these activities will result in significant risk reduction.[3]

The early guidelines offered by grassroots organizers were sensible, logical and based on a good epidemiological model generated by gay men with an understanding of the range of sexual behaviours and institutions in their community. It remains solid advice. But many people, including leaders in AIDS organizations, were uncomfortable with this advice until doctors lent their stamp of approval. Condoms in particular were a source of equivocation. In the US, the Federal government is largely culpable here; for a long time they refused to fund direct research on the efficacy of condoms. Even after HIV was identified, they said no technology existed to test condoms for HIV permeability. Finally, in the summer of 1986, some California researchers constructed an ingenious device consisting of plungers to which condoms could be attached. Their studies showed that even under extreme conditions, the virus did not pass through the latex.

Today public discourse on AIDS focuses on condoms for heterosexuals. Little mention is made of the now longstanding use of condoms by gay men.

'Whatever You Want To Do, You Can Probably Do It Safely'

It has been hard for many people to hear the safer sex message. Despite the best intentions of AIDS activists, safer sex guidelines are often perceived as limiting or judgmental. This is largely due to the conflation of sexual practice and sexual identity in US culture. Gay men often initially feel that eliminating a central sexual practice means they are 'no longer gay'. In addition, sex is perceived as the cement in the gay male community: many gay men fear that if sexual rites are reduced or de-emphasized, the community will lose its unique identity and disintegrate.

Despite the complex elements that form our sexual identity and community, the safer sex message is about sexual practice and is quite simple. It was eloquently stated by a gay man with AIDS who is a safer sex educator: 'Whatever you want to do, you can probably do it safely'. That means continuing activities that do not involve exchange of semen and blood, and under some circumstances, faeces, urine or saliva, if there is reason to believe quantities of blood may be in them. When you engage in activities where these fluids have direct access to absorptive tissues like anal and vaginal tissue, or abrated tissue, like open cuts in the mouth or hands, then you should use barriers like condoms, surgical gloves, or dental dams. It is that simple.

But the public AIDS discourse equates condoms and/or celibacy with safer sex, ignoring the wider range of safer sex practices. Negative attitudes toward condom use (and in many cases, toward celibacy) and the erroneous idea that only 'at risk' people need to practice safer sex seems to promote a risk perception logic that encourages the reader to identify with the categories of *people* identified as 'not at risk' rather than looking at their own sexual and drug use *behaviours* to determine what changes might be necessary. Thus, a man who does not identify as gay, but who engages in sex with another man might decide categorically that he is not 'at risk' and does not need to change his behaviour. His identification of 'not at risk' preempts the assessment process that is really the hallmark of the safer sex package.

Women especially have difficulty applying safer sex information couched in the 'safer sex = condoms' equation because they often already have difficulty negotiating sex with their male partners. Merely popping on a condom or abstaining shifts neither the power dynamics nor the lack of attention to the nuances of pleasure that both gay liberation and feminism criticized in heterosexualist sexual practice. If sex is to be shifted away from high-transmission activities and retain a strong erotic attraction, it must address the social and psychological attitudes that already problematize sex for everyone but the most intransigently heterosexual.

The ultimate problem with this pared down message about safer sex is that it leads people to the conclusion that risk assessment is best accomplished by taking the HIV-antibody test. It leads to the assumption that risk reduction is based on antibody status, and reduces the responsibility for change to the level of individual protection rather than the transformation of group mores and expectations.

The elaborateness of gay male sexual culture which may have once contributed to the spread of AIDS has been rapidly transformed into one that inhibits the spread of disease, still promotes sexual liberation (albeit differently defined), and is as marvellously fringe and offensive to middle America as ever. Heterosexuals in the US, who do not as often participate in an articulate sexual culture, may initially experience few opportunities for exposure to HIV but also have fewer experiences of sexual community that can provide the locus for transformation to safer sex values. Women, for example, in the absence of a strong women's movement, must fight their battle for safer sex on the carefully guarded and privatized domain of relationships with individual men. Gay men can find empowerment among a community of men who demand the practice of safer sex. Safer sex norms will ultimately be more difficult to achieve among heterosexuals than in the urban gay world. The history of women and birth control does not give cause for optimism about the ability of heterosexual culture to achieve safer practices that respect all partners involved.

The Attack on Promiscuity

Perhaps the single most misunderstood 'fact' about the transmission of HIV is that promiscuity is the chief culprit. Despite wide media and even scientific reporting, epidemiological studies show that it is not primarily number of sexual partners, but rather exchange of infected semen or blood that creates risk for contracting the virus. Number of partners is significant only to the extent that those practices involve an exchange of semen or blood through a direct route — anally or vaginally, or through cuts in the hands or mouth. Conversely monogamy *per se* doesn't decrease risk if one or the other partner is HIV antibody positive or transmits an as yet undetected co-factor during unsafe sex. Even those who accept this reality often argue that monogamous relationships provide a better context for discussing risk history and preferred methods of risk reduction. Studies of gay men however show that coupling does not necessarily produce more discussion of safer sexual practices. They show that men give the same reasons for not practising safer sex whether they are in a monogamous relationship, a primary relationship with occasional other partners, or involved in primarily anonymous sex. Indeed, in the sexual economy of the baths, bars, or bushes, it may be much easier to refuse a sexual encounter with an unreformed stranger than to deal with safer sex with a reluctant long-term lover with whom one shares more complicated relationship issues.

Safer Sex may be Hazardous to Women

While it is unequivocally true that women are more likely to acquire than to give HIV infection when having sex with a man — thus requiring more 'protection' — monogamy and condom use as promoted in the media are fraught with danger.

The current technology for AIDS risk reduction and the fact that no major campaign has insisted on the responsibility of heterosexual men (as opposed to the campaign to protect one's self from prostitutes, a transmission link that is not demonstrable) mean that women must ask men to wear condoms. Women exist in a sexual economy where they have unequal power in relationship to potential sex partners; this inhibits their ability to make a risk evaluation and reasonable changes. While some gay men complain of boredom or loss of gay identity when they try to practise safer sex, many women fear their sexual partner's responses to their safer sex requests. In addition, because heterosexuality proposes fewer activities that count as 'real sex' (fucking is the model, as opposed to the wider range of activities articulated in urban gay male culture), women find it difficult to direct their male partners away from the hazardous activity of intercourse.

Successful safer sex education for women depends on politicizing women about the same issues feminists raised in dealing with birth control: a woman's right to choose how she will use her body and men's obligations to take responsibility for sex.

In this era, when most birth control is designed to exist hidden inside a woman's body, people in the age groups most affected by AIDS have never had to negotiate male-centred contraception. This is strongly reflected in the condom marketing campaigns. By several counts, women now comprise 70 per cent of the condom buying market in the US. If we consider that gay men constitute a large percentage of the remaining condom buyers, we can only conclude that heterosexual men represent the greatest stumbling block in heterosexual safer sex.

Safer Sex is Sexual Liberation

Safer sex describes specific practices that prevent the hazardous exchange of infected or possibly infected body fluids. It is not a moral category to sweep up sexual practices with which we feel uncomfortable for other reasons. Gay sex can be safer. S/M can be safer. Anonymous sex can be safer. Bisexual sex can be safer. Monogamy in itself is not safer, and, though a valid option for any number of reasons, carries its own dangers — spouse abuse and all the traditional hazards of 'marriage'. Celibacy prevents the spread of HIV, but carries its own psychological hazards.

Safer sex should be a key agenda item for progressives, but it must be pursued in a context that gives control over how the safer sex message is articulated and how safer sex norms are enforced. It is hard to persuade those who do not yet engage in safer sex to do so if the state continues to have the power to arrest people for sodomy. It is hard to promote self-esteem when lesbians and gay men are declared categorically unfit as parents or teachers. It is hard to talk about the experience of AIDS when jobs and homes can be lost for 'coming out' or for being perceived to be linked with AIDS. Even heterosexual people have suffered 'gay' oppression when they are linked with AIDS — recently a woman lawyer was detained, strip searched, and forcibly tested when she was found to be in possession of condoms.

Vessels and Vectors: Losing the Battle Against Testing

Until there was wide discussion of AIDS among heterosexuals, gay and AIDS activists had held the line against widespread testing. There were currents of dissent, including those who believe that a knowledge of test results increased behaviour change, a position that is disputed. Research projects measuring changes made by those who know and those who do not clearly fail to support this contention.[4] Until recently gay activists, civil libertarians, and AIDS activists were quite successful in controlling how and when the test was used. In the US, as concern increased (or was displaced) onto pregnant women and 'innocent victims' about to be married, testing policy headed down the slippery slope of medical abuse.

This was primarily because the Right occupied the corner of the AIDS discourse that concerned women and children. Feminists had not taken AIDS or HIV testing on as an issue, and gay men had ignored, or been too busy to recognize, that the social control of women in American society is still so keenly sought by the Right that the testing of women would become the linchpin in the plan to test and isolate those infected with HIV.

The fact is that women, described by the Right and many epidemiologists as the 'vector' for moving AIDS between communities, have long been viewed as the reservoir of disease. Further, women are the 'vessels' of procreation, which gives men an additional stake in controlling their bodies. If you believe that women (read: prostitutes) are spreading AIDS to nice men who then take it home to their wives (vessels for producing the next generation), then it makes a certain perverse sense to demand the HIV testing of women. If you imagine that gay men are a hermetic community (that is, no straight men get their virus while engaging in homosexual acts) then who cares if they take the test? There are a plethora of right wing and left wing rationalizations for letting gay men decide for themselves but forcing women who intend to have sex and children to be tested against their will.

Evolution of Testing Ideology

In 1984, the US announced the development of a test for the antibody to the recently identified HTLV-III — the putative AIDS agent. CDC and the National Institutes of Health (NIH) officials advocated early widespread testing — even before the test was through its trials, and despite the fact that it had no diagnostic value. It did not show who would get AIDS or ARC and who would not, who was infectious and who was not. Moreover, the test had been designed to accept a high false positive rate as a trade-off for decreasing the number of false negatives. Early estimates placed the false positive rate at 10 per cent to 30 per cent. Subsequent protocols augmented the so-called ELISA test with the more expensive Western blot, but at the time of initial calls for mass testing, the test protocol to be used had a very high false positive rate. No one knew the exact incubation period for the virus. At that time, estimates were five to seven years. No one knew the length of time between initial infection and the production of antibodies.

Certainly, the wish to prevent any more suspect blood from entering the blood supply prompted quick government action. But it is important to remember that at the time testing became feasible, CDC and NIH officials widely believed that transfusion and blood products were the principal route of transmission from gay men and injecting drug users to the 'general population'. Foisting the test on risk groups thereby gave society at large a sense that something was being done — and only these unpopular groups would suffer the ramifications of testing. Testing was in place, and large numbers of people had been tested before a full policy analysis of the effect in insurance, civil liberties, individual mental health, and general health actions could be determined. There have clearly been disastrous side-effects for the minority communities perceived to be 'at risk'. Testing lulled people who perceived themselves to be members of the 'general population' into believing AIDS was being effectively addressed, that a vaccine and cure were around the corner, and that their status outside the 'risk groups' would ensure their safety.

AIDS activists and gay leaders moved quickly to discredit the testing programs. Citing not only the problems with the test and the psychological impact of those tested, they argued that at least those testing positive would be at risk for losing insurance (insurers had already tried to claim AIDS was a pre-existing condition, and in some cases, claimed it was an 'elective' illness), jobs, housing. Some feared that positive test lists would leak from agencies and might be used to 'round up' people for quarantine, legally harass prostitutes, or merely expose anyone who sought the test as gay or a drug user, statuses not protected under most civil rights laws.

The US government countered these concerned by offering to fund anonymous sites called, in true government doublespeak, 'alternative test sites'. In addition, at the request of health activists, testing was mandated to take place with pre- and in some cases post-test counselling and referrals. Although a few major AIDS organizations attempted to block the creation of the alternative test sites in their areas (notably, Chicago and Philadelphia), most took the attitude that sites would be created anyway, and that AIDS groups should cooperate in their creation in order to control their subsequent activity.

At this time, most AIDS groups strongly counselled against test taking. At best they saw alternative test sites as a way to get the state to pay for AIDS activists to talk gay men out of taking the test. Groups in Chicago and New York produced material for wide public distribution that admonished 'don't take the test'. Soon, however, some gay activists began to argue that it was good to take the test, that men would change their behaviour. Properly designed record systems could assure the confidentiality of those taking the test — a claim made in the face of at least four documented cases of government agencies 'accidentally' releasing test lists. Some went so far as to accuse anti-test activists of irresponsibility in counselling against taking the test. The ethics argument soon devolved into a contention that 'anyone has a right to take the test' and that it was possible to counsel people in such a way as to obtain meaningful consent. Few included the possibility of civil rights infringements in their attempts to gain 'consent'.

The media misunderstood or misrepresented the HIV-antibody test from the start, and, within months it became known as 'the AIDS test'. Testing gained tremendous credibility, and news reports represented AIDS organizations as offering a much needed service by providing testing. The counselling style changed substantially from an attempt to talk people out of taking the test to offering 'only the facts'. The gay run alternative test sites ceased to be a ruse for getting government money to carry out health education at a time when no money for this was officially available.

When the CDC, in late 1985, requested proposals for the first health education dollars, it mandated that testing must be incorporated into education, implying that they would only accept projects where the educational process centred around testing. The National Coalition of Gay STD Servics, health care providers and even some CDC officials objected to this emphasis on testing rather than education. AIDS groups were nervous about using the test before its psychological and legal effects were known, and some CDC officials were concerned about mixing seroepidemiological data gathering and educational projects. At the time, those who favoured testing asserted that knowledge of status was pedagogically effective. But in time, the serosurveys would become part of the epidemiology literature and test sites would be pressured to incorporate blind serosurveys. These retro-fitted serosurveys would become an evaluation tool of the original educational projects.

Consequences of Taking the Test

Some people feel their anxiety will be relieved by being tested. This is true for some people, but the test often raises as many anxieties as it quells. In one study, many men expected to test positive and were negative. Far from being relieved and returning to a 'normal' life, they increased stress-outlet behaviours like binge drinking and drug abuse. They expressed feelings of survivor guilt toward sick friends or lovers. About a third of these men became hooked on testing, going back for many repeat tests and living in consistant anxiety between test results. In couples tested together, a HIV antibody negative partner sometimes broke up with an HIV antibody positive one. If both were HIV positive, they often tried to assess blame, assuming one had infected the other, even when both could have been infected independently.

Ultimately, individuals decide whether it makes sense for them to take the test. But it should be a rigorous part of the 'informed consent' process that everyone understands the wide range of psychological responses and legal hazards of the test.

The Obligation to Know

The Reagan administration is fond of claiming that people have a moral obligation to know their test status and should be legally culpable for behaviour after being so informed. This is a wrongheaded way to make people take responsibility for their behaviour.

There are continual cases of HIV antibody positive people being accused of attempted murder for spitting on or biting someone. This is a ruse to arrest HIV antibody positive people or further detain HIV positive prisoners for events and actions unlikely to transmit the virus. At the present time, the state would rather spend money on testing to define who should be rounded up than spend money on health education. Education could teach people that they cannot contract AIDS by being spat upon by others. Education could teach about the thirty-odd people recorded as having been bitten by institutionalized patients with AIDS who did not acquire HIV infection.

There are other cases of people prosecuted for attempted murder for having sex with a partner who subsequently decided that the accused knew or *should have known* that they were HIV antibody positive. This says that people who test positive are responsible for making sure safer sex is practised, but people who are negative are not. The idea that one has a moral obligation to know rests on the wish to believe that only those who are HIV antibody positive need change their behaviour. It comes from the mistaken idea that if only the HIV antibody positive people could be isolated, AIDS would go away. Notions like this ignore a much simpler method of isolating the virus: putting a little latex between sexual partners of either status.

The Hidden Agenda: Racism and Classism

With new testing mandates, the Reagan administration — and its New Right constituency — is testing the waters for future measures like quarantine. Further, the effects of widespread testing on women are at cross-purposes with the reproductive rights movement agenda of the last fifteen years. Testing pregnant women can only lead to forced sterilization and forced abortion (long-time opponent of abortion, Surgeon General C. Everett Koop, now concedes that HIV antibody positive status is a condition under which abortion should be available to women). Women with HIV infection give birth to HIV antibody infected babies in about 20–40 per cent of cases. New research suggests that the probability of *in utero* infection varies with the degree of infection of the mother. While women who are at risk may well want to get tested in order to help them make a child-bearing decision, it does not make sense for all pregnant women to be tested. If women intend to have the baby anyway (and certainly, we grant women in this society the right to carry out high risk pregnancies) or if they will consider abortion if they are already pregnant, then the test can only be an anxiety-producing event which yields little useful information.

The agenda behind required testing of all pregnant women is racist and classist. The plain fact is that the majority of women with AIDS in the US are black (50 per cent), with a large number of Hispanic woman (20 per cent) and only about a quarter white (27 per cent). Half are injecting drug users, and a quarter more are the non-injecting partners of drug-using men. Children who contract HIV infection *in utero* are disproportionately children of colour. The numbers reveal why testing poses such dilemmas for communities that are rightly suspicious of limits or restrictions on conception. A New York physician and researcher who works with these women said to his colleagues at the June 1987 International AIDS Conference in Washington, DC, that his clients' biggest problems were food and shelter, not the results of their HIV antibody tests. Even Koop has now joined the ranks in opposition to mandatory testing of pregnant women, on the grounds that it would cut down on access to pre-natal care among women who believed they may be at risk. Mandatory testing of these women, irrelevant to the real conditions of their lives, only compounds the obstacles they already face in terms of jobs, housing and access to services.

Making Sexual Choices

Taking the test will not settle personal fears about AIDS. Neither will it cause AIDS to disappear. Allowing the test to be widely used will not solve the present health crisis. AIDS is with us as a disease and a social phenomenon, and will not go away no matter how many people take tests. AIDS has changed our concept of sexuality by heightening our fears and requiring us to talk about and plan our sexual activities, something that makes many Americans very uncomfortable. The media's crass summary of the situation is that we should just stop having sex outside of marriage.

The message is especially troublesome for women, who have long been told they cannot make good choices about sex. The message we must take from AIDS is that we *can* choose wisely, and we can protect the health of ourselves and our partners. But the choice should not be based on a test result; it should be based on understanding how transmission occurs and on taking the simple steps to avert it. The message is to expand our concept of sex, to increase the discussion of pleasurable possibilities, and to eroticize measures that reduce transmission of *all* sexually transmitted diseases.

Notes

1 This chapter is dedicated to Bob Andrews, Boston, MA, gay and civil rights activist for a decade and a half, and AIDS activist from 1982 until his death from AIDS in March 1988. Bob and I shared much of the history described here, and his comments and perspective were crucial to the chapter's realization.

2 Some of these trained bar-tenders as educators, and involved zap actions where leather-clad hunks raided bars to pass out condoms and literature.

3 Data from the project were presented at the 1987 Lesbian and Gay Health Conference in Los Angeles.

4 Data relating to this were recently summarized in the National Institutes of Health report at the February 1987 conference on HIV Testing. A preliminary report published by the National Institutes of Health in April 1987 concluded that in studies of gay men and injecting drug users, knowledge of antibody status in itself did not provide predictable behaviour changes. Moreover, data from the study of gay men in Baltimore presented at the 1987 Lesbian and Gay Health Conference in Los Angeles showed no difference in sexual behaviour between those learning their antibody status and those who did not. Data from San Francisco shows slightly higher adherence to sexual behaviour changes in those learning their antibody status. Unfortunately, many of these studies have used number of partners as the significant marker of behaviour change, rather than the incidence of high-risk transmission activities.

References

BERKOWITZ, R., CALLEN, M. and DWORKIN, R. (1983) *How to have Sex in an Epidemic*, News from the Front Publications, New York.

FOUCAULT, M. (1984) *The History of Sexuality Volume 1*, Harmondsworth, Penguin Books.

RUBIN, G. (1984) 'Thinking sex: Notes for a radical theory on the politics of sexuality', in VANCE, C. (Ed.) *Pleasure and Danger*, London, Routledge and Kegan Paul.

16
Reading AIDS

Jan Zita Grover

The season of AIDS is upon us, as anyone passing a newstand, browsing through a bookstore, or cruising the airways via remote-control knows well. Unhappily, the majority of book titles in the 1987/88 US winter–spring listings on AIDS are clustered at one end of the spectrum of possible approaches to this most complicated of cultural and scientific phenomena — these are the guides on how-to-avoid-AIDS and how-to-have-safe-but-exciting-sex. Their number is seemingly legion, and their range is from uptight-conservative to adventurous-liberatory.

Clustered at the other end of the spectrum are books that treat AIDS as a subject of history. They seek to place the legal, political, media and medical dimensions of AIDS alongside other cultural phenomena and assess its impact on them, their impact on it. The most conspicuous title in these terms is Shilts' (1987) *And the Band Played On*, a 613-page (excluding its 16-page index) novelization of the epidemic from its traceable origins in the mid-1970s to the death of Rock Hudson in the summer of 1985, with a coda on the opening of the Third International Conference on AIDS in Washington, DC, in summer 1987.

Shilts' book has won widespread and generally unqualified praise in mainstream US media, in large part because Shilts' values and techniques are its own. Certainly the book is a *tour de force* of organization; it moves backward and forward in time and space in byte-sized pieces portentous of the growing epidemic. The personal stories of epidemiologists, politicians, research scientists, physicians, gay activists, PWAs (people living with AIDS) — and many of Shilts' subjects pass through more than one of these categories — are spliced into each other. Like a restive channel-switcher, Shilts aims at a simultaneity of action.

While *And the Band Played On*'s initial effect is dazzling in its sheer intricacy, eventually I found it counterproductive. Television and *USA Today* may have conditioned large audiences to ten–second bites of information and analysis, but I want and expect more from a history — particularly a 613-page history with few precedents.[1] The flashy technique used here produces ironies by the gross, as contiguity invariably does, but irony is not a satisfying substitute for analysis, and it is analysis that this book sorely lacks.

Geoffrey Stokes, in his review of *And the Band Played On* in the January/February 1988 issue of *Columbia Journalism Review*, remarked that Shilts' account 'is rather too quick to impute evil motives, too slow to give weight to the huge inertial factor built into any large bureaucratic institution'. Though Stokes singled out Shilts's condemnation of media's inadequacies — inadequacies having 'as much to do with (media's) standard operating procedures as with the conscious, or even unconscious, homophobia Shilts finds' — the same is true of the shortcomings of political, public-health, and medical institutions. These too failed, as Shilts demonstrates, but their failure cannot simply be said to be caused by, as he claims they are, homophobia.

Let us concede first of all, that until recently politicians, whether gay or straight, conservative, liberal, or radical, have not been deeply engaged in matters of sexually transmitted diseases, other than to deal with them repressively — as Allan Brandt (1985), in his splendid *No Magic Bullet: A Social History of Venereal Disease in the United States since 1880* makes convincingly clear. Let us concede, furthermore, that injecting drug use is a social issue that in the past has excited little political interest other than continuous confusion over the differences between *preventive/treatment* measures such as education, counselling, methadone or other options and *encouragement.* Concern for the latter can be seen in the action of politicians like US Senator Jesse Helms who sees an acknowledgement of these issues as tantamount to condoning them. Similarly gay activists did not widely organize around the rising incidence of hepatitis B, herpes virus, and other sexually transmitted diseases in gay communities in the 1970s and early 1980s.

The stage was thereby set for dealing poorly with both sexually transmitted diseases and injecting drug use — the primary routes by which HIV is transmitted in the US. AIDS in America, then, was born into a political and operational climate, particularly with Reagan's unconstrained budget-slashing in 1981/82, that made a slow and conservative institutional response almost an inevitability.

There are problems beyond Shilts' relatively crude analysis of institutions, however. Part of the allure of the book to the entertainment industry, I suspect (the book was immediately bid up for television and film by 20th Century Fox-TV and other Hollywood institutions), is the familiarity of the tactics it uses to solicit reader response; this is the tried-and-true tale of history's heroes, a neo-Emersonian narrative of selected individuals who have Made A Difference. Among these, as practically everyone knows by now, is Patient Zero, a French-Canadian airline steward whom Shilts first alleges conceivably brought AIDS to the US — and then goes on to produce a highly coloured, fictionalized account of this very 'fact'. As source for this information, Shilts cites the 'cluster study' conducted by William Darrow of the US Federal Centers for Disease Control (CDC). Darrow, as Duncan Campbell (1988) reported, recently repudiated Shilts' use of that study and the inferences Shilts drew from it, which depend for their plausibility on progression from initial HIV infection to clinical AIDS of only nine–eleven months, whereas it is now clear that the average incubation period is more like seven-and-a-half years. Moreover, Shilts's reliance on the strategy of reading history exclusively through individuals embeds analysis in personality — in the people selected to highlight events, and in the statements selected to personify them. This makes an analysis of institutions exceptionally difficult. In true American fashion, it views them predominantly as the constructs of individuals like Anthony Fauci of the National Institute of Health and Don Francis (then) of the Centers for Disease Control. Such a method, while dovetailing perfectly with the approach of popular news and entertainment, reduces the complexity of institutional responses to the attitudes and behaviours of a few selected members of these organizations. Quite simply, the ways organizations respond to any challenge are more complex than such an analysis can allow.

And the Band Played On is, as the blurbs would have it, a book that cannot be ignored. The public should know how tail-dragging, how territorial, its own public agencies are — the shameful record of the White House in this respect, happily, speaks for itself. Shilts' painstaking reconstruction of the US blood-banking industry's resistance to HIV antibody-screening also is important for us to know and condemn. The public also should know that key public-health agencies, like more ideologically transparent institutions, are as politically and culturally bound to certain values and practices as the church or the school. Science as a pragmatic study — the great fantasy/desire of nineteenth-century middle-class progressives — needs to be put in a political perspective: it is no more objective or empirical than Roman Catholicism or supply-side economics. For identifying the limitations to this vision, Shilts is to be congratulated.

At the same time what his history *leaves out* profoundly mis-shapes what remains: as Rose Appleman detailed in her review of *And the Band Played On*,[2] Shilts' account does not point out that by 1982, AIDS was affecting minority communities and injecting drug users — the urban poor already most affected by other sexually transmitted diseases, tuberculosis, and malnutrition — and for whom AIDS was yet another instance where the US healthcare system failed. Likewise, although lesbians in San Francisco and New York were among the first people to help care for gay men with AIDS, both inside and outside AIDS service organizations, there is no evidence of their contribution in Shilts' account. By 1985, when Shilts ends his narrative, AIDS had become a major problem (as well as a series of attempted political and organizational solutions) to a far wider cross-section of Americans than middle-class white gay men. But one could not know that from Shilts' story. This does not mean that the partiality of his account reduces its value: it simply misrepresents that value. *And the Band Played On* is a fairly narrow, even parochial account, and it would have been more accurate, less arrogant, to have presented it as such.[3]

The other notable title to appear recently on the cultural/political AIDS front is Yale University's excellent *AIDS and the Law*, an anthology of pieces written (most of them successfully) for non-lawyers on a wide range of topics: AIDS and the military, the schools, housing, physical handicaps, prisons, employment, medicine, and other social institutions. The preface, a short course on law for the layperson, is a wonderfully clear exposition of the bases for legal process and a step-by-step description of a hypothetical AIDS-related civil case. That and the excellent chapter on the differences between medical and legal cultures and the inevitably antagonistic relations of physicians and lawyers are invaluable for *any* reader, much less someone engaged in dealing with the many legal precedents, actions, statutes and ordinances that comprise our codified dealings between individuals and institutions.

But meanwhile, back in the realm of popular non-fiction, all is not so clear, so civil. A recent spate of books, culminating in the release of Masters, Johnson, and Kolodny's (1988) hysteria-mongering *Crisis: Heterosexual Behavior in the Age of AIDS*, assure their anxious publics that AIDS is now upon them. Most of them aim, if implicitly, at an average, poorly-defined middle American — white, middle-class, sexually not very adventurous or promiscuous (and by the latter term I mean nothing derogatory). Such texts — which include Art Ulene's (1987) *Safe Sex in a Dangerous World*, and Helen Singer Kaplan's (1987) *The Real Truth About Women and AIDS* make large assumptions about the identity of their readers, pushing black and Hispanic people to the edges of their arguments as uniformly high-risk individuals, and identifying gay men and lesbians as entirely beyond the pale of their concern.

Rather than emphasizing *risk reduction*, as gay safer-sex advocates have sought to do, these authors stress *risk elimination* through HIV antibody testing. 'Say *no* to him until he is tested and cleared', Kaplan advises her women readers, recommending the use of the 'Lysistrata strategy' to them — no sex with *any* man unless he is tested. This piece of advice, incidentally, is the only remotely collective action advocated by any of these authors — sex and politics for them is an atomized drama taking place in isolated, individual bedrooms nationwide, not something that people can discuss and organize around. '(I)t is nonsense to speak of "avoiding unsafe sexual practices". All sexual practices are safe with an uninfected man', Kaplan states. And then, revealing the central message of these deeply conservative books, she equates clearing-by-testing with a return to the longed-for past: 'You can throw away those annoying condoms, diaphragms, and smelly jellies and disinfectants'. Did people dispense with them entirely before the AIDS epidemic, as Kaplan seems to imply? Ah, the bygone golden years, when pregnancy, herpes, and other STDs were supposedly loved and familiar threats — those years onto which we can project our present longings, our longed-for simplifications, without any fear that they will speak back! The HIV seronegative, if they test themselves obsessively enough, wash thoroughly enough, can ride out the epidemic as if it simply were not happening.

We can not make sense of the call for widespread HIV antibody testing in most of these books unless we understand the profound distrust and veiled contempt their authors feel for the sexual (and social) experience of their readers. For authors like Kaplan and Ulene, testing is a liberatory activity because it 'frees' men and women to resume previous sexual activities secure in the knowledge that they are 'safe' from HIV infection. Only constant monitoring, however, can eliminate the possibility of infection, for in Kaplan's and Ulene's deeply misanthropic views, lying, dissimulation, and evasion are normal *modus operandi* among heterosexual men, who are, moreover, interested only in their own pleasure and generally poor lovers. Kaplan includes a number of imaginary scenarios in which her (female) reader negotiates safer sex and/or the demand that her partner be tested. Significantly, none of these concludes with the man actively resisting the request. Though his doing so is implicit in everything else Kaplan says about men *vis-à-vis* AIDS, such a reaction was evidently too nettlesome to consider within the confines of a book that sees testing as the sole solution to virtually every HIV-related problem. But anxiety will out: a great deal of obsessive energy is displaced onto long-shot possibilities of transmission via the male body: 'Do not let him come anywhere *near* your pubic hair or genitalia . . . that whole area is moist when you are excited and the AIDS bugs can 'swim' right into your body that way. You must wash immediately and disinfect the place where his semen wet you'.[4]

I find it remarkable how consistently misanthropic these stridently heterosexist books, written by and for women, are. Kaplan and Ulene are also dismissive and contemptuous of gay men, Kaplan going so far as to speculate that it is gay men protecting their own interests who have caused federal and local government agencies to devise 'AIDS-related health legislation' that is 'at best inadequate and in fact actually *destructive* to women and children'.[5] The inconvenient fact that it was the large gay-male AIDS organizations in New York and San Francisco, Gay Men's Health Crisis and the San Francisco AIDS Foundation, that produced the first publicity on women and AIDS goes by the board here; Kaplan is not dealing in facts so much as prejudices. Such power, of course, is always attributed to one's scapegoat. In the real world beyond Kaplan's paranoia, however, gay power in the US has moved precious few legislative mountains; until very recently it has, instead, turned inward toward its community crisis and focussed primarily on work within the voluntary sector.

At the most fundamental level, these texts deny the lived experience of those for whom they claim to be written. Kaplan in particular appears to write in a social vacuum. A physician and sexologist, she is so far removed from grasping the simple facts of transmission via blood transfusion that she suggests, 'donating blood is an excellent way of getting tested for free if you have any doubts about *your AIDS status*'.[6] Kaplan has clearly never visited a blood-banking site and worked her way through its elaborate system of self-screening questions, a process that would void such a suggestion. Neither would she appear to have learned anything about the risk to the blood-supply of high-risk donations outlined in such damning detail in *And the Band Played On*.

Both Kaplan and Ulene emphasize the 'dangers' of condoms because they are not 100 per cent effective in preventing pregnancy and, by implication, the transmission of HIV.[7] But it is evident from their discussions that both favour monogamous relationships, view multiple sex-partners as evidence of moral laxity or immaturity, and see women as *essentially* more monogamous, less sexually engaged, than men: 'Women do not mind monogamy and sexual exclusivity as much as gay men do; in fact, many prefer sex in a committed relationship. Women as a group have always been more interested in the *quality* of sex rather than *quantity* provided by different partners'.[8] Quite apart from the fact that women *as a group* have never been united in their sexual preferences (much less anything else), her imaginary group betrays Kaplan's own values, which are socially and sexually conservative. We are to be congratulated, she tells us, upon the fact 'that AIDS has put an end to casual sex with strangers, "but I don't consider this a loss. In fact to me, the one silver lining in the dreadful AIDS cloud is that people will have to get to know each other better and develop an intimate, trusting and caring relationship before they have sex. *Most women have always wanted good sex with one beloved man* rather than a number of partners".'[9]

This kind of emphasis upon an all-or-nothing-at-all approach to sexual relations in the age of AIDS ignores the facts of sexual and marital relationships in the US and other Western societies: few people mate for life, and HIV testing far from constitutes the perfect marker of infection that Kaplan and Ulene sees it as, particularly among the newly infected and persons in low-risk populations.[10]

Ulene's, Masters, Johnson and Kolodny's, and Kaplan's texts are grossly overbalanced in the direction of sexual 'what-ifs' and exceptional cases. Everything else gets short shrift, including issues of AIDS and race: 'black and Hispanic women are especially vulnerable. If you are in *one of these situations* you are definitely at risk.'[11] Women as *social beings*, as care-givers, as drug users, as lesbians involved in gay politics, as users of artificial-insemination, are completely ignored in these accounts. These texts contain no discussion of the spectrum of health, financial, and social problems of HIV-infected women or women diagnosed with AIDS. In a peculiar way, these conservative books also fashion heterosexual men and women as exclusively sexual beings: AIDS has no meaning beyond the perils it poses in selecting and coupling with a sexual partner. Moreover, one could have no idea in reading them that both men and women have organized collectively around the AIDS epidemic, both to serve people living with HIV infection and to help prevent it within their own communities (in the absence of much except obstruction on the part of the US government).

In a strange way, these texts are also stunningly American. The solutions they propose are wholly individual, they derive what authority they possess from their authors' professional credentials as physicians,[12] and they see prevention lying in a technological fix — the HIV-antibody test — rather than in collective and individual efforts to modify behaviour. Prudish in the extreme, Ulene repeatedly invokes ovulation as an analogue of HIV infection,[13] Kaplan despatches anal sex with the claim 'The anus was not designed for sexual purposes',[14] and they all aim to return 'the general population' to a sexuality it never enjoyed in the first place.[15]

The most frightening thing about books like those by Kaplan, Ulene, and Masters, Johnson and Kolodny is that they are being distributed and marketed by major publishers. This almost guarantees them wide sales and credibility as well as secondary media exposure via television. Kaplan and Ulene have been repeatedly interviewed as 'AIDS experts', and Masters, Johnson and Kolodny alone have been effectively challenged for their conclusions on Ted Koppel's *Nightline.*

A number of far more humane and useful texts on safer sex have been produced this year for (primarily) heterosexual women — Chris Norwood's (1987) useful *Advice for Life*, Cindy Patton and Janis Kelly's (1987) *Making It*, and Diane Richardson's (1987) *Women and AIDS*, first published in 1987 in Britain as *Women and the AIDS Crisis*, and now updated with more US material. Each of these books treats HIV infection and AIDS as part of a larger picture than the bedroom, which the other texts discussed here do not. AIDS and HIV clearly affect women and men at many levels besides the sexual, and these books discuss them.

Norwood, Patton and Kelly, and Richardson consider AIDS to be both a social and personal issue. Norwood's discussion of sexual practices, her recommendations for risk reduction and the range of issues she addresses are far broader than those of the medics discussed above. She makes more (and more intelligent) use of epidemiological and clinical studies than any of the other authors, including the physicians, and extends her coverage to discuss HIV infected but asymptomatic women, women after diagnosis of AIDS and ARC, the dilemma of infected women with children, and women as care-givers. Nevertheless, while she is more compassionate and complex in her treatment of women and AIDS, she still portrays gay men as whipping-boys. For example, she suggests that in sounding out a (male) partner for possible risk-factors, a woman might say, 'I'm sure you know that people are worried about AIDS. I think we should talk about it . . . even a guy who shot up drugs a few times *or got seduced by some guy when he was a teenager* might have a small risk.'[16] No harm in that — we all know that gay men are seducers and that a heterosexual man can only be *the object* of another man's desire!

Patton and Kelly pack an extraordinary amount of information into their short bilingual (Spanish and English) text. The range of their discussion is light-years beyond that of the physicians, and is politically savvier and more compact than Norwood's. It is grounded in a recognition of many kinds of drug and sexual practices. It is succinct, often humorous, and absolutely non-judgmental in discussing practices that either excite condemnation or go entirely unmentioned elsewhere — S/M sex, sex-for-hire, anal and vaginal fisting. Their practical suggestions on minimizing risks while performing these activities, described in blunt and descriptive language, are a model for preventive education. In twenty-five pages, they also cover the pros and cons of HIV antibody testing, risks during pregnancy, artificial insemination and lesbian safer-sex. Perhaps most important, both the text and the accompanying drawings by Alison Bechdel address the interplay between individual decision-making on women's parts and the possibilities for group action, group learning and support about AIDS.

Richardson's *Women and AIDS*, intended as a more comprehensive guide, is equally generous in its tone and more extensive in its range. Safer sex — again based on the principles of risk reduction rather than risk elimination — is dealt with carefully and at length. There are chapters on the epidemiology of HIV infection in women, including HIV and drug use, rape, prostitution; risks to African and Haitian women; lesbians and AIDS; living with HIV infection, AIDS and ARC; woman as care-givers (discussed within a feminist perspective on women's unpaid work); and a chapter on AIDS public policies and prevention.

These three texts see gay men's hard-won insights into risk-reducing sexual practices as models of political and personal practice, experience painfully and heroically gained, and experience, moreover, that demonstrably *works*.[17] In contrast, Kaplan, Masters, Johnson and Kolodny, and Ulene rebuke or dismiss the experience and safer-sex expertise of gay men, offering their own abstract formulas instead.[18]

It is not often that we are present at the birth of a cultural phenomenon, placed in a position to watch the ways it is first woven of words and acts. AIDS is as much a creation of language as it is of the body or of love and fear. The words that are used to expand or set limits on our understanding of it must be attended to closely. These books, setting out to define Americans' relation to AIDS, are variously mean and generous, hopeful and pessimistic, practical and speculative. Thankfully, their readers will not engage with them in a vacuum but within the framework of their prior experiences of health, sickness, desire, sexual, gender and social identities, politics and history. Even the nastiest of these texts contains some useful information and provides opportunities for thought.

I am optimistic about Americans' attitudes towards AIDS because I see evidence in public-opinion polls, as well as in the beliefs and actions of people around me, that AIDS is always viewed and interpreted *within discrete communities* — which are, after all, where each of us lives our daily lives. Here, AIDS is not seen monolithically or reductively, but complexly and dynamically. The opposing view — that 'heterosexuals' (which ones?), are terrified of AIDS, that 'people' (what people?) generally behave with extraordinary viciousness toward children infected with HIV[19] — is the confection of those same media sages who bring us 'the general population' and humankind reductively constructed for purposes of profit as age-sex-household income-habits of consumption. Unlike these crude media models, lived experience makes each of our encounters with AIDS immensely complicated — it forces us to confront what we think we know and why we think we know it.

Notes

1 The two exceptions in English are Altman's *AIDS in the Mind of America* (New York, 1985) reprinted as *AIDS and the New Puritanism* (London, 1986) and Patton's *Sex and Germs: The Politics of AIDS* (Boston, 1985). Both are better-balanced accounts than Shilts'; their limitation is simply that of their positioning in time, approximately two years before Shilts completed his account.

2 'AIDS exposé paints vivid picture — but watch out for what's missing', *Frontline* (Oakland, CA), 15 February 1988, pp 6–7.

3 Readers of San Francisco's monthly gay and lesbian newspaper, *Coming Up!*, have commented negatively on Shilts' treatment of many of these same issues in their recent letters to the editor; see for example, 'Homosexual Zero: Randy Shilts' letters from Tim Burak, John D. Dolan, and Lon

G. Nungesser in *Coming Up!*, May 1988, pp 2–3.
4 Kaplan (1987), p 111.
5 *ibid*, p 39.
6 *ibid*, p 103.
7 *ibid*, p 71 'If (a woman) relies on a condom instead of the test, she could die if some infected fluid from his moist pubic hair touches her genitalia'.
8 *ibid*, p 46. Emphasis here on *women as a group* is mine: the rest is hers.
9 *ibid*, p 49, emphasis added.
10 Serological and epidemiological data thusfar suggest that the average length of time between exposure to HIV to an infection that produces detectable anti-HIV antibodies is between three weeks and six months. There have been studies, however, that indicate it may take as long as eighteen months for some persons to produce detectable antibodies. In low-risk populations, the number of false-positive HIV antibody tests is unacceptably high, given the political, economic and social consequences of seropositivity. On the other hand, the number of false-negatives in a high-risk population is much smaller. Antibody testing may soon be rendered moot and a new phase of testing begun when Polymerase Chain Reaction (PCR) testing becomes commercially available. This testing replicates any vital protein present in a sample until it is measurable. HIV is present before measurable amounts of HIV antibody.
11 Kaplan (1987) p 98, emphasis added. Tell this to a middle-class American black or Latino and see what sort of reaction you get.
12 It is significant, I think, that the admirable Cindy Patton-Janis Kelly and Diane Richardson texts discussed below are written by people active in the gay-lesbian and feminist health communities, where lack of a medical degree is not seen as a barrier to responsible theory and practice on health issues. These authors' authority derives from their first-hand experience with HIV/AIDS counselling and activism. Significantly, none of the 'medical experts' — Masters, Johnson and Kolodny, Kaplan, Ulene — has an HIV-AIDS medical practice or is an AIDS activist, unless one defines the latter as a book contract and publisher-sponsored lecture tour.
13 Ulene (1987) p 24: 'Unlike fertility, there is no "safe" period with respect to transmission of the AIDS virus'; 'It is important to note that there is no "safe" period during which the AIDS virus is absent, unlike the "safe" period that occurs with respect to fertility' (p 58).
14 Kaplan (1987) p 80.
15 Here the spirit of the late Raymond Williams can be heard to whisper, 'An idealization, based on a temporary situation and on a deep desire for stability, serve(s) to cover and to evade the actual and bitter contradictions of the time' (Williams, R. (1985) *The Country and the City*, London, Hogarth Press, p 45).
16 Norwood (1987) p 57, emphasis added.
17 For example, the incidence of new seroconversions among the cohorts of gay men observed in San Francisco's long-term prospective studies in 1987 was less than 1 per cent. Researchers conducting those studies for the San Francisco City and County Department of Public Health, the University of California-San Francisco, and San Francisco General Hospital acknowl-

edged at the Department of Public Health's monthly Grand Rounds in February 1988 that credit for this marked decline in new HIV infections was not due to 'saturation of the herd' or public-health measures, but to gay men's collective and individual actions. See also Morin, S.F. (1988) 'Behaviour change and prevention of sexual transmission of HIV' (abstract), IV International Conference on AIDS, Stockholm, p 368.

18 See Patton's critique of this pattern among latter-day, self-appointed 'AIDS experts' elsewhere in this book.

19 US media have made a great deal of the trials of HIV infected children in Florida and Indiana who were made pariahs in their hometowns, and of the man in West Virginia who was burned out of his home. As of 16 May 1988, over 60,000 persons in the US have been diagnosed with AIDS, the majority of them not having been burned out, shot at, or totally shunned. What interests are being served (and compensated for) in mainstream media's emphasis on the atypical, the extreme, and what are the connections between 'the typicality of the extreme' and the 'typicality of the common' otherwise invoked in the media's representations of 'the general population'?

References

ALTMAN, D. (1986) *AIDS and the New Puritanism*, London, Pluto Press.

BRANDT, A. (1985) *No Magic Bullet: A Social History of Venereal Disease in the United States Since 1880*, New York, Oxford University Press.

CAMPBELL, D. (1988) 'AIDS: A new history and a new myth', *New Statesman*, 2971, pp 22–3.

KAPLAN, H. S. (1987) *The Real Truth About Women and AIDS: How to Eliminate the Risks without Giving up Love and Sex*, New York, Fireside Books/ Simon and Schuster.

MASTERS, W., JOHNSON, V. and KOLODNY, R. (1988) *Crisis: Heterosexual Behavior in the Age of AIDS*, New York, Grove Press.

New Statesman, (1988) 4 March.

NORWOOD, C. (1987) *Advice for Life: A Woman's Guide to AIDS Risks and Prevention*, New York, Pantheon.

PATTON, C. (1985) *Sex and Germs: The Politics of AIDS*, Boston, MA, South End Press.

PATTON, C. and KELLY, J. (1987) *Making It: A Woman's Guide to Sex in the Age of AIDS*, Ithaca, NY, Firebrand Sparks Pamphlets.

RICHARDSON, D. (1987) *Women and the AIDS Crisis*, London, Pandora Press.

SHILTS, R. (1987) *And the Band Played On*, Harmondsworth, Penguin Books.

ULENE, A. (1987) *Safe Sex in a Dangerous World: Understanding and Coping With the Threat of AIDS*, New York, Vintage Books.

Notes on Contributors

Peter Aggleton is Principal Lecturer in Education Policy Studies at Bristol Polytechnic. He is Director of the Young People's Health Knowledge and AIDS Project, the Learning About AIDS Project and the Learning about AIDS Young People's Project. He is the author of *Nursing Models and the Nursing Process* (with H. Chalmers, Macmillan, 1986), *Deviance* (Tavistock, 1987), *Rebels without a Cause?* (Falmer Press, 1987) and the editor of *Social Aspects of AIDS* (with H. Homans, Falmer Press, 1988).

Lindsey Alldritt is a researcher with the Monitoring Research Group at Goldsmiths' College, London.

Mary Boulton is Lecturer in Medical Sociology at St Mary's Hospital Medical School, London. Her research interests include the health beliefs and health behaviour of gay men in response to AIDS, and the sexual identity and sexual behaviour of bisexual men. She is the author of *On Being a Mother* (Tavistock, 1983) and *Meetings between Experts: An Approach to Sharing Ideas in Medical Consultations* (with D. Tuckett, C. Olsen and A. Williams, Tavistock, 1985).

Stephen Clift is Senior Lecturer in Educational Studies at Christ Church College, Canterbury. He is the Co-director (with D. Stears) of the HIV/AIDS Education and Young People Project.

Peter Davies is Senior Lecturer in Social Sciences at South Bank Polytechnic. He is the Co-director of Project SIGMA (Socio-sexual Investigations into Gay Men and AIDS) and author of *Key Texts in Multidimensional Scaling* (Heinemann, 1982) and *Images of Social Situation* (Sage, 1985).

Kate Dolan is a researcher with the Monitoring Research Group at Goldsmiths' College, London.

Martin Donoghoe is a researcher with the Monitoring Research Group at Goldsmiths' College, London.

Ray Fitzpatrick is University Lecturer in Medical Sociology and a Fellow of Nuffield College, Oxford. His research interests include the health beliefs and health behaviour of gay men in response to AIDS, and the sexual identity and sexual behaviour of bisexual men. His publications include *The Experience of Illness* (with J. Hinton, S. Newman, G. Scambler and J. Thompson, Tavistock, 1984).

Ronald Frankenberg is Professorial Research Fellow in the Centre for Medical Social Anthropology at the University of Keele. His publications include *Communities in Britain* (Penguin Books, 1966) and *Custom and Conflict in British Society* (Manchester University Press, 1982). His current research interests include medical anthropology and the study of children affected by the three epidemics.

Jan Zita Grover edits a data based textbook on HIV infection at San Francisco General Hospital. She has published widely on AIDS and has recent articles in *October* and the *Women's Review of Books.*

Graham Hart is Lecturer in Medical Sociology at University College and Middlesex School of Medicine, London. His research interests include the health beliefs and health behaviour of gay men in relation to AIDS, the health behaviour of bisexual men in response to AIDS and an evaluation of a needle exchange scheme in central London. He has recently contributed chapters to *Caring for Health: Dilemmas and Prospects* (Open University Press, U205, 1988) and *Readings for a New Public Health* (edited by C. J. Martin and D. V. McQueen, Edinburgh University Press, 1988).

Meyrick Horton is an AIDS Programme Officer with the Health Education Authority. He has been involved in AIDS organizing since 1983. Prior to his present appointment, he was Health Education Officer for the Terrence Higgins Trust in London. His current research interests include the formation of an AIDS Research Paradigm and its relationship to education and social policy.

Geraldine Mulleady is Senior Clinical Psychologist at St Mary's Hospital Drug Dependency Centre, London. She has worked in the clinic for four years and is responsible for HIV and drug services. She is involved in the management of the Syringe Exchange Unit and has acted as a consultant to the World Health Organization on HIV-related counselling issues and drug abuse.

Cindy Patton is a journalist who has been involved in AIDS organizing for six years. She is the author of *Sex and Germs: The Politics of AIDS* (South End Press, 1985) and *Making It: A Woman's Guide to Sex in the Age of AIDS* (Firebrand Press, 1987).

Robert Power is Research Officer at the National Institute for Social Work, London. Between 1985 and 1988, he was Research Fellow on the Drug Indicators Project at Birkbeck College, London. His current research interests lie in the field of fields of dementia amongst the elderly and the abuse of illicit drugs. He has published widely on issues to do with drug use and has contributed chapters to *Socialism in a Cold Climate* (edited by J. A. G. Griffith, Allen and Unwin, 1983) and *Drugs and British Society* (edited by S. MacGregor, Tavistock, forthcoming).

David Silverman is Reader in Sociology at Goldsmiths' College, London. He is the author of *The Theory of Organisations: A Sociological Framework* (Gower, 1970), *Qualitative Methodology and Sociology* (Gower, 1985) and *Communication and Medical Practice: Social Relations in the Clinic* (Sage, 1987). His current research interests focus on the counselling of people with HIV infection and AIDS.

David Stears is Senior Lecturer in Educational Studies at Christ Church College, Canterbury. He is the Co-director (with S. Clift) of the HIV/AIDS Education and Young People Project.

Gerry Stimson is Principal Lecturer in Sociology at Goldsmiths' College, London and Director of the Monitoring Research Group. His research and teaching interests are in the sociology of health and illness, and social responses to drug problems. His publications include *Heroin Addiction: Treatment and Control in Britain* (with E. Oppenheimer, Tavistock, 1982).

Simon Watney is Chair of the Social Policy Group of the Terrence Higgins Trust in London and was a researcher on the Learning about AIDS Project at Bristol Polytechnic. His research interests lie in the field of higher education, sexuality and photography. He is the author of *Policing Desire* (Comedia/Methuen, 1987).

Jeffrey Weeks is a social historian and sociologist with research interests in the social regulation of sexuality. His publications include *Coming Out* (Quartet, 1977), *Sex, Politics and Society* (Longman, 1981 and 1989), *Sexuality and its Discontents* (Routledge & Kegan Paul, 1985) and *Sexuality* (Tavistock, 1986).

Tina Wiseman was Health Education Officer with the Terrence Higgins Trust in London. She is currently a consultant to UNICEF in connection with their HIV and AIDS education programme in Kenya.

Index

ACT UP (AIDS Coalition to Unleash Power) 72, 226
active-passive ratio 157–8
ADAPT (Association for Drug Abuse Prevention and Treatment) 206
Advice for Life (Norwood) 259, 260
Advisory Council on Misuse of Drugs 11
Africa
  denial of epidemic in 27
  heterosexual transmission in 88–9
  HIV in heterosexuals 26–7
  regional patterns 26–7
age
  behaviour change and 137–8
  knowledge and 138
Aggleton, Peter 74–100, 199–210, 220–36
AIDS
  1981–82, dawning crisis 3–4
  1982–85, moral panic 4–6
  1985 onwards crisis management 6–8
  as sexually transmitted disease 76–80
  as social phenomenon 25
  as vulnerability 33, 67
  association with marginal populations 3, 9
  perceptions of sufferers 70–1
  permissiveness link with 12
  perverse nature of 80–5, 87
  social response 2, 13–15
  tests *see* HIV-antibody tests
Aids: A Guide to Survival 31
AIDS and the Law 255
AIDS week (1987) 42
AIDS-Related Conditions (ARCs) 65, 66
Alma Ata Declaration 21
Amsterdam 200
  syringe exchange 190
And the Band Played On (Stilts) 252–5
Anne, Princess Royal 17, 26
anonymous/alternative test sites 246, 247
anti-gay backlash 12
anxiety 106, 109–10, 121–2
Appleton, Rose 255
ARCs *see* AIDS-Related Conditions (ARCs)
Asia, regional patterns 28
attempted murder charges 248
Australasia 24–6
Australia, health education in 30
AVERT 167
awareness 131
AZT *see* clinic case studies

Baldwin, James 17
behaviour change
  gay men *see* gay men behaviour change
  injecting drug users 174, 181–2, 200–1
Black Community AIDS Team 217
blood supply contamination 7, 86
Bloomsbury Health Authority 165
Body Positive 25, 34, 226
Boulton, Mary 127–46
Boyson, Sir Roydes 12
Brandt, Allan 253

Index

Campbell, Duncan 254
Canadian Laboratory Centre for Disease Control 86
Carribbean, regional patterns 26–7
CDSC *see* Communicable Diseases Surveillance Centre (CDSC)
celibacy solution 149, 239
Center for Disease Control (Atlanta) 24, 76, 238
Central London Action on Street Health (CLASH) 165
chastity 80
children *see* innocent victims
China 22
Chinese Community Health Care Centre 217
cholera 10
Christian doctors 16
Christians and AIDS 47, 51
CLASH *see* Central London Action on Street Health (CLASH)
class *see* social class
Clift, Stephen 39–63
clinic case studies 101–26
  desire for secrecy 106–7
  doctor behaviour 116–17
    avoidance of psychological issues 117–20, 121
  experienced patients 104–5
  infection and identity 105–7
  need to be responsible and trustworthy for doctors 114–16
  patient behaviour *see* patient behaviour
  presentation of self 107–14
  setting 102–4
  social organization of care 123–4
  staff division of labour 123
  staff present 103
Communicable Diseases Surveillance Centre (CDSC) 161
community care 33
  contributions from users and ex-users 207
  family support counselling 207
  injecting drug users 206–7
community issues 17–18
community-oriented health education 223, 224, 226, 229, 231–2
compulsory testing 14, 16, 27, 32, 68, 71
  pregnant women 249
  women 245
contagious diseases 66, 71
control *see* locus of control
costs, of gay men behaviour change 136–7
counselling 32, 97, 196, 207
crisis management 6–8
Cuba 22, 27
cultural natural selection 94–5
cultural theory, AIDS and 64–73

Dannemeyer, Congressman 72
Darrow, William 254
Davies, Peter 147–59
death, social acceptance 31–3
dementia 23, 35, 65, 66
Dingwall, R 105
discrimination 22, 34–6
  employment 57
divine retribution 26, 47, 51, 67
doctor behaviour 116–17
  avoidance of psychological issues 117–20
Douglas, Mary 124
Drug Injectors Project (Birkbeck College) 174
drug users *see* injecting drug users
drugs
  denial on cost basis 31, 72
  paying to be guinea pigs 72

Eastern Europe, regional patterns 28
Economic and Social Research Council (ESRC) 147–8
Edinburgh 162, 163, 164, 176, 177, 187, 189, 191
education, safer-sex *see* safer sex education
ELISA test 245
employment disccrimination 57
ethnic minorities 258
  health education for 212, 213
  HIV testing 249
ethnographic enquiry 95, 97
evaluation of health education 227–34
  attitudinal 227
  behavioural 228
  choice of evaluators 232–5
  cognitive 227
  community-oriented model 229, 231–2
  holism 233–4

information-giving education 228, 230–1
outcome evaluation 227–30
process evaluation 230–2
self-empowerment education 229, 231
expenditure
cutting commitment of New Right 10–11
denial of drugs on cost basis 31, 72
experienced patients 104–5

family 69
enobling of 79
perceived threat to 79
support 33, 207
FAO 21
Fauci, Anthony 254
fear 87
see also moral panic
financial difficulties 206
Fitzpatrick, Ray 127–46
Flynn, F 90–1
Foucault, M 64, 69, 83
Francis, Don 254
Frankenberg, Ronald 21–38
Frontliners 105, 110, 112, 226

Gallo, Robert 76
Gay Bar Syndrome 86
Gay Bowel Syndrome 86
gay cancer 4
gay men
1981–82 awakening anxiety 3–4
analysis of sexual activity *see* homosexual sexual activity analysis
anti-gay backlash 12
attitudes to 57
backlash against 12
behaviour changes *see* gay men behaviour change
communities 17–18, 84
decontamination rituals 5
self help response 6
social arrangement variations 81–2
success of safer sex 67
gay men behaviour changes 127–46
age and 137–8
cost and benefits 136–7
knowledge and 131–2, 142
locus of control 132–5
private lifestyle groups 134, 135, 137
public lifestyle group 134
regionally derived cultural differences 133
risk perceptions 129–30, 142
social class and 137
social support 135–6
support groups and normative values 238
testing and 138–40, 246
Gay Men's Health Crisis 6, 257
gay plague 4, 5
Gay Related Immune Deficiency (GRID) 85
gay rights, drop in support for 12
genital herpes 9
germ theory of medicine 75
Glasgow 163, 176, 177
syringe exchange schemes 187, 196
Greater London Youth Matters 217
GRID (Gay-Related Immune Deficiency) 4
Grover, Jan Zita 252–63
guilty parties 17, 35, 80

haemophiliacs 3, 26
Haitian community 3, 4, 76, 86
Hart, Graham 127–46, 160–72, 199–210
Health and Social Security, Dept of 189
publicity campaign 29–30, 223–4, 227, 228
Health Belief Model, behaviour change and 136–7
health education
Australia 30
Britain campaigns 24, 29–30, 223–4, 227, 228
community participation 212
community-oriented model 223, 224, 226, 229, 231–2
Danish campaign 29–30
DHSS campaign 223–4, 227, 228
different models of 222–4
ethnic minorities 212, 213
evaluation *see* evaluation of health education
information-giving model 214, 215, 221, 222–4, 228, 230–1
language difficulties 213
marginalized groups and 211–19

objections to safer-sex education 72
offensive language 53
participatory approach 224
people with learning difficulties 213
self-empowerment model 214–15, 222, 223, 225–6, 229, 231
shower and bidet dissemination models 215–16
socially transformatory model 223, 226, 232, 239–40
Terence Higgins Trust 216–18
top-down and bottom-up initiatives 214–15
young people 213
see also safer sex education
Health Education Authority 24, 234
Health Education Council 24, 234
health improvement teams 167–8
health outreach work 164–6
injecting drug users 204–5
health services, expenditure cutting 10–11
hepatitis 9
heroin users *see* injecting drug users
heterosexual transmission 94
early discounting of 87–90
in Africa 26–7
HIV 23, 76
dormant 65
identification of 5
latency period 23, 66
suggested African origins 27
see also HIV antibody tests
HIV antibody tests 66
anonymous/alternative sites 246, 247
as sole solution 256–7
behaviour change and 138–40, 246
civil rights and 247
compulsory 14, 16, 27, 32, 68, 71, 244–5, 249
consequences of 139, 247–8
ELISA test 245
evolution of ideology 245–6
high false positives 245
injecting drug users *see* injecting drug users
legal effects 246
obligation to know 248
punitive *see* compulsory testing
racism and classism 249
HIV induced dementia 23, 35, 65, 66
homophobias 71
homosexual sexual activity analysis 147–59
abstention 149
active-passive ratio 157–8
coding 151–3
end sequences 153–5
grammar 149–51, 155–6
indexicality 150
orgasm as end marker 153–4, 158–9
Project SIGMA 147, 148
role-specificity 155–7, 158
homosexuality
changing political climate on 13
defined as disease 15, 16, 82–3
limiting promotion of 12
unnatural 12
see also gay men: homosexual sexual activity analysis
Horton, Meyrick 74–100
hospice care 207
housing problems 206
How to Have Sex in an Epidemic 239
Hudson, Rock 6
Human Immunodeficiency Virus *see* HIV

immigration control 27
India 22
individual protection 242
infectious diseases 66, 71
information giving 214, 215, 221, 222–4, 228, 230–1
injecting drug users 26, 160–72, 203–4
AIDS as motivation for seeking help 181–2
behaviour changes 174, 181–2, 200–1
community care 206–7
cultural variations 178–9
epidemiology 161–2
ethnic variations 178–9
family support counselling 207
gender variations of infection 187
geographical distribution of infection 162
harm minimization strategies 173, 183, 199–210
health improvement teams 167–8
HIV infection levels 161–2, 187
HIV testing 203–4
housing and financial difficulties 206
infection source to heterosexual population 169

initial identification of risk 4
initiation 207
levels of risk 199–200
methadone treatment 201–3
method of drug use 173–85
needle and syringe availability 47, 163–4, 183, 187–8
needle exchange schemes 166–7, 175–6, 183
outreach work 164–6, 204–5
police attitudes 163–4, 176–7, 188, 189, 192, 197
prevention programmes 207–8
regional variations 177–8
self-help 205–6
sexual risks 201
sharing circumstances 162–3, 174–5, 179–80
situational context 180–1
social and behavioural aspects of transmission 162–4
sub-cultural differences 164
syringe exchange schemes *see* syringe exchange schemes
innocent victims 17, 26, 33, 53, 80
children 79
international issues 16–17, 21–2, 23
isolation *see* quarantine

Johnson, V 256, 259, 260
journals 94, 96
Junkiebonden 206

Kaplan, Helen Singer 256, 257, 258, 259, 260
Kaposi's sarcoma 76
Kaunda, President 27
Kelly, Janis 259, 260
knowledge
age and 138
behaviour changes and 131–2, 142
endorsement or acceptance 132
Kolodny, R 256, 259, 260
Koops, Dr CE 7

latency period 23, 66
Latin America 27
Leicester YMCA 217
Lesbian and Gay Centre Youth Project (New York) 240
lesbians
backlash against 12
community issues 17–18
decontamination rituals 5
drop in support for 12
self help response 6
lifestyles
private 134, 135, 137
public 134
literature
medical texts 94, 96
publications 252–63
Liverpool 163, 177
syringe exchange scheme 191, 192, 193–4
Local Government Act (1988) 12
locus of control
behaviour changes and 132–5
personal efficacy 133–5, 142
response efficacy 133
London Declaration 22, 23, 28
London Lesbian and Gay Switchboard 220
London Weekend Television 12

Maccario, M 90–1
McClelland Committee 189
Mahler, Hafdan 23–4
Making it (Patton and Kelly) 259, 260
Management of AIDS patients, The 31
Manchester 181
Mann, Jonathan 23
marginalized groups, health education and 211–19
Masters, W 256, 259, 260
medical texts 94, 96
medico-moral issues 15–16
methadone treatment 201–3
Michigan study *see* Multicentre AIDS Cohort Study
Middle East 28
Monitoring Research Group (Goldsmiths' College) 174–5, 192
monogamy 80
Montagnier, Luc 76
morals
moral panic 4–6, 71, 87
traditional 234, 239
undergraduates' attitudes 56–60
volume of hatred and contempt 69–70
Mort, Frank 1–2
Mulleady, Gerry 199–210

Multicenter AIDS Cohort Study 128, 130, 133, 135, 139, 141

National Bureau for Handicapped Children 217
National Coalition of Gay STD Services 247
National Institute for Health (Bethesda) 24
National Institutes of Health 245, 246
needle exchange schemes 166–7, 175–6, 183
  see also syringe exchange schemes
neurological disorder 23, 35, 65, 66
New Left, AIDS and 14
New Right
  crusade against permissiveness 11–12
  expenditure cutting commitment 10–11
  moral politics of 9–13
  welfarism and 13–14
No Magic Bullet: A Social History of Venereal Disease in the United States since 1880 253
normative beliefs, behaviour change and 135–6, 142, 238
Northern Road Drug Clinic (Portsmouth) 202
Norwood, Chris 259, 260

objective behaviour 110–11, 122
offensive language 53
ostracism 34–6
outreach work 164–6
  injecting drug users 204–5

Pacific region 28
Padgug, Robert 6
Padian, Nancy 88–9
panic *see* morals, moral panic
parasitic disease 90
passivo-activo complex 82
patient behaviour 104–5
  anxiety 109–10, 121–2
  cool style 108–9, 120–1
  need to be impress doctors 114–16
  objective style 110–11, 122
  positive thinking 112–14, 123–4
  presentation of self 107–14
  theatrical style 111–12, 122
patients
  denial of expensive drugs to 31, 72
  living with AIDS 30–1
  perceptions of 70–1
Patton, Cindy 8–9, 14, 237–51, 259, 260
Pearce, Richard B 89–90
People with AIDS coalition 72
permissiveness, link with AIDS 12
personal efficacy, behaviour change and 133–5, 142
Pneumocystis carinii pneumonia 76, 85
police attitudes 163–4, 176–7, 188, 189, 192, 197
Polk, B. Frank 87–8
Popek, E 90–1
positive thinking 112–14, 123–4
Power, Robert 173–85
pregnant women, compulsory testing 249
prevention 23, 28–30
  see also health education: safer sex education
professionalization 8, 14, 237–8
prognosis
  after test 66
  uncertainty 32–3
Project SIGMA 147, 148
promiscuity 242–3
promotion of homosexuality limitation 12
psychological issues, doctor avoidance of 117–20
public lifestyle group 134

quarantine 14, 16, 28, 36, 57, 249

racism 258
  HIV antibody tests and 249
  see also ethnic minorities
Reagan, President Ronald 7, 10, 12
Refuge Action 217
regional patterns 24–8
responses
  professionalization of 8
  self help 6
research paradigm 74–100
  discourse regulation arena 96–7
  early discounting and heterosexual transmission 88–9
  scientific thought styles 92–5
  texts 94, 96
respite care 207

response efficacy, behaviour change and 133
Richardson, Diana 259, 260
risk, generalization of 7
risk behaviour 26, 35, 67, 86
risk categories 10, 26, 35, 67, 86
  initial identification of 4
  see also gay men: injecting drug users
risk perception 241
  behaviour changes and 129–30, 142
  denial of virulence and 129–30
role-specificity 155–7, 158

safer sex 25, 40, 47
  success in gay community 67
safer sex education 6, 237–45
  gay community and 237–9
  objections to 72
  overprofessionalization of 8, 14, 237–8
  responsible advice 239–40
  risk perception 241
  safer sex as liberation 244
  sexual identity and community 241
  see also HIV antibody tests
St Mary's Drug Dependency Unit 199, 204, 205, 206
San Francisco AIDS Foundation 257
San Francisco Men's Health Study 128, 133, 141
SCODA *see* Standing Conference on Drug Abuse (SCODA)
Scottish Home and Health Department 189, 190
secrecy, desire for 106–7
section 28 12
segregation *see* quarantine
self help
  alternative health care and therapies 8
  initial organization 6
  organizations 25, 28, 34, 52–3
  pressure groups or service agencies 14
  professionalization 14
  welfare dependence on 14
self-empowerment health education 222, 223, 225–6, 229, 231
sexual activity
  behaviour changes *see* behaviour changes: gay men behaviour changes
  diversity 69–70
  neurophysiological basis of 91
  sexuality 69–70
  social tensions and 9–10
  see also homosexual sexual activity analysis
sexually transmitted disease 35
  identification of AIDS as 76–80
  social evils 1
Sheffield syringe exchange scheme 191, 194
Shilts, Randy 7, 17–18
Sigma *see* Project SIGMA
Silverman, David 8, 16, 101–26
Small, Neil 2
smallpox 21
Smallwood, Gracelyn 30
social care *see* welfarism
social class
  behaviour change and 137
  HIV antibody tests and 249
social diseases 1
social hygiene movement 79–80
social ostracism 34–6
social response 2
social support, behaviour change and 135–6
socially transformatory health education 223, 226, 232, 239–40
Socio-sexual Investigations into Gay Men and AIDS *see* Project SIGMA
Sontag, Susan 1, 106
South East Thames Regional Health Authority 40
Soviet Union 22, 28
Standing Conference on Drug Abuse (SCODA) 220
Stears, David 39–63
stigmatization 22
Stilts, R 252–5
Stimson, Gerry V 166, 186–98
Stokes, Geoffrey 253
sub-group alienation 211–12
support groups 33
  behaviour change and 135–6, 142
  changing normative values 135–6, 142, 238
  complementary 34
  family 33
  Frontliners 105, 110, 112
  peer group behaviour 206
  self help and individual groups eg.

Terrence Higgins Trust
symbolic significance 2, 9–10
syndrome, distinction between virus and 65
syphilis 77–8
syringe exchange schemes 47, 166–7, 176, 183, 190–2, 204
  ability to attract clients 193, 195, 197
  Amsterdam 190
  background 186–8
  counselling quality 196
  funding 11
  Glasgow 187, 196
  lack of public opposition 196–7
  legal issues 188, 192
  Liverpool 191, 192, 193–4
  location of 195–6
  national and regional variations 187
  numbers of syringes issued 191, 194
  police reactions to 188, 189, 192, 197
  policy changes 188–90
  preliminary assessment 195–7
  progress with 192–3
  Sheffield 191, 194
  staff 191, 195
  traditional availability 188
  user-friendliness 195
  see also injecting drug users: needle exchange schemes

Terrence Higgins Trust 6, 25, 216–18, 220, 226
testing *see* HIV antibody test
textbook science 94, 96
Thatcher, Margaret 10, 12
theatrical behaviour 111–12, 122
thought-styles 92–5
  intellectual leaders 92–4, 95
transmission, heterosexual *see* heterosexual transmission
treatment
  care without cure 32
  counselling 32
  denial of expensive drug treatment 31, 72
  hospice care 97
  prolongation of life 30–1
  see also counselling

Treichlker, Paula 5
typhoid 10

Ulene, A 256, 257, 258, 259, 260
undergraduates' beliefs and attitudes 39–63
  anticipated outcomes 43–4
  changes between surveys 60–1
  data collection 42–3
  elementary linkage analysis 53–6
  item correlations 53–6
  questionnaire 41
  religious and non-religious students 59–60
  results of questionnaire 47–53
  sample 44–5
  sex differences 45–7
  worry and moral attitudes
  student characteristics and 57–60
  summated scales concerned with 56–7
UNESCO 21
United States 24–8
University College Hospital Drug Dependency Clinic 168
unnatural practices 12

venereal disease *see* sexually transmitted disease
virus, distinction between syndrome and 65

Watney, Simon 64–73, 124
Weeks, Jeffrey 1–20, 101–2
welfarism
  fiscal crisis of 13
  New Right and 13–14
WHO 21–2, 27
Wiseman, Tina 211–19
Wolfenden Report 83
women
  compulsory testing 245
  lack of group support 242
  need for male-centred contraception 243, 245
  pregnant, compulsory testing 249
Women and AIDS (Richardson) 259, 260
Women and the AIDS Crisis (Richardson) 259, 260
World Health Organization 190, 212